The
Tai Chi
Healing
Bible

The Tai Chi
Healing Bible

A step-by-step guide
to achieving physical and
mental balance

Mark Green

APPLE

A QUANTUM BOOK

This edition published in 2014 by
Apple Press
74-77 White Lion St
LondonN1 9PH

ISBN: 978-1-84543-528-8

Produced by
Quantum Publishing Ltd
The Old Brewery
6 Blundell Street
London N7 9BH

QUMTAIB

Assistant Editor: Jo Morley
Editors: Hazel Eriksson and Sam Kennedy
Consultant Editor: Mark Green
Production Manager: Rohana Yusof
Publisher: Sarah Bloxham

Packaged by Gulmohur

Printed in China by Midas Printing
International Ltd.

Quantum would like to thank and
acknowledge the following for supplying the
pictures reproduced in this book:

Shutterstock: p6, 7,9, 11, 12, 18, 41, 46, 62,
    85, 86, 98, 111, 131, 145, 153, 158, 178,
    179, 181, 183, 189, 191, 192, 197, 200,
    202, 203, 205, 206, 207, 210, 211, 213,
    214
iStock: p18, 36, 48
Alamy: p10
Getty: p14
Corbis: p15

All other photographs and illustrations are the
copyright of Quantum Publishing Ltd

While every effort has been made to
credit contributors, Quantum would like
to apologize should there have been any
omissions or errors.

The material in this book originally appeared
in *Tai Chi A Practical Introduction* and
Tai Chi for Mind, Body & Spirit.

Contents

Introduction

The first time I realised there was something seriously wrong with my left knee I was 13 years old. Bone disease and cartilage damage led to my first surgery aged 16, then again at 18, 20 and 23. By that time I found myself sitting in a London hospital in the company of a world famous knee surgeon. With a grave face he told me that, even if I convalesced, my knee would last, at best, 18 months. Then the inevitable full joint prosthesis would follow. That was 18 years ago and I still have the same left knee I had that day. How is this possible? Because of Tai Chi.

Some years earlier I happened to meet a Tai Chi Master. I had been fascinated with Martial Arts since I was a child, growing up with Bruce Lee and the arrival of Hong Kong action movies in the West. I explained my situation to the Master and he turned to me and said, 'Tai Chi will heal your knee.' Just a simple statement, but he said it with such gravity and conviction I couldn't possibly doubt. So I started to train.

So much damage had already occurred to my knee that it took years of dedicated practice before real improvement happened. But it did, and it continued until, aged 30, I gave up a career in medical research to teach Tai Chi full time.

So how does it work? Much research has been done showing how Tai Chi affects the cardiovascular, nervous and respiratory systems. Your blood becomes more oxygenated. Your circulation is improved. Bone marrow is enriched and immune function increases. Breathing techniques massage internal organs. Slow movement assists venous return taking pressure off your heart. Moving meditation relieves stress and anxiety. The list goes on. Traditional Chinese Medicine describes how Tai Chi improves the flow of Chi energy through the acupuncture meridians. Clearing blockages and restoring balance and, consequently, good health. These are not familiar concepts to us in the West but don't worry, the way to understand Chi is to experience it. With time and practice all Tai Chi students report sensations of warmth in their hands and feet, tingling in their fingertips, a magnetic feeling between their palms, a new found sense of wellbeing. The ancient Chinese masters that crafted this art had the same experience and simply described it as 'the energy of the body moving', Chi!

The more you practise, the more you will relax. The more you relax, the more you will feel your Chi. Some people experience this in their first lesson. For others it can take months. Practising Chi Kung as well as Tai Chi helps a lot.

The best way to learn Tai Chi is with a good teacher. If one is not available to you, *The Tai Chi Healing Bible* will really help to get you started. The Yang twenty-four Tai Chi Form taught in this book is a great place to begin. If you have found a teacher and have started to learn the twenty-four-step Form I also highly recommend this book. One of the biggest barriers to progress in the first few years of Tai Chi is simply memory. Having a good reference text is a great help. In addition to the Tai Chi Form this book also shows you many excellent Chi Kung Exercises. In contrast to Tai Chi, Chi Kung is very easy to learn. One of its great strengths is its simplicity. I am confident you will be able to teach yourself some good Chi Kung easily from this book. I hope *The Tai Chi Healing Bible* will give you an excellent introduction to Chinese healing arts.

Below The steps followed when practising the Tai Chi Form progress from one to the next with great fluidity.

Good luck with your training

Dr Mark Green

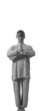
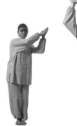
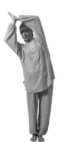
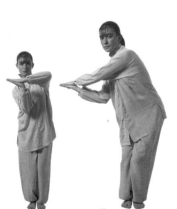
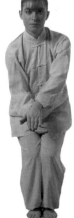

Origins and Principles of Tai Chi

What is Tai Chi? As you learn more about Tai Chi, your definition will change. Your perceptions will lean more toward one aspect of the art at different times.

As an exercise, put down this book now and, on a blank piece of paper, define in your own terms what YOU perceive Tai Chi to be. You description can be as direct or as abstract as you like, as long as they mean something to YOU. This is a useful exercise that should be done several times as you develop your skills and personal understanding of Tai Chi.

It is true that trying to define Tai Chi can never be totally accurate – as the Taoists have said for many years, the essence of a thing is un-nameable, and it is easier to describe what a thing is not, rather than what it is. It is, however, a useful exercise and reference point.

Right Tai Chi sword: There are many portals through which you can approach Tai Chi. In the past, one of the most common was through the study of the martial arts.

Fundamentally Tai Chi stems from three cores of Chinese knowledge, which are:
(1) Martial arts
(2) Healing arts
(3) Philosophy

As a martial art, Tai Chi employs softness rather than strength. This can be likened to the flexible strength of a willow tree that bends and twists in a storm, compared to the rigidity of a great oak tree, which can be uprooted and blown over.

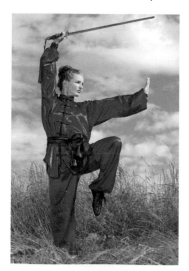

8

Redirecting Energy

An example of this flexibility is yielding to re-direct a force rather than meeting it head-on. The re-direction will require very little physical effort whereas the head-on approach would need a greater force to neutralise the oncoming force. Therefore using softness means that the strongest force will not necessarily win every time.

This is the meaning of the classic Tai Chi phrase, 'use four ounces to deflect a thousand pounds'.

With time and practice you will begin to experience and understand the energy aspects of Tai Chi. Gradually your energy levels will increase. Excess energy is accumulated in the body and can be used for any of the various healing arts or martial arts practice.

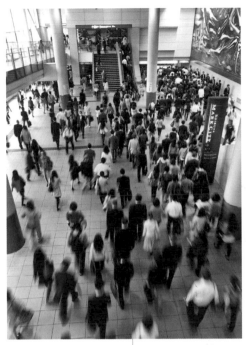

Above Tai Chi's unique combination of exercise for the mind, body and spirit is the ideal antidote to the stresses of modern life.

Behind the overall frame of Tai Chi, lies an understanding of the Universal forces of Yin and Yang. While many people have seen the black and white Yin/Yang symbol, fewer are aware that it is actually called the Tai Chi symbol. By practising Tai Chi, you can learn about Yin and Yang through direct experience, rather than a theoretical knowledge gained from a book.

There is another quality of Tai Chi that should never leave us – it is fun. There should always be this kind of a soft enjoyment to your Tai Chi practice, which, when observed, will not look intimidating to children.

Tai Chi has many different angles of exploration. There are various styles of Tai Chi, and even different ways of doing the same style. Within any one style there will usually be elements of form (pattern) training, energy-building and self-healing exercises (chi kung), martial applications and combat training methods, pushing hands and weapons training.

Remember – learning Tai Chi should be fun!

Tai Chi Legends

The origins of Tai Chi have become clouded in the mists of time. There are various explanations as to where it originated, many of them involving legendary Chinese alchemists or Taoists.

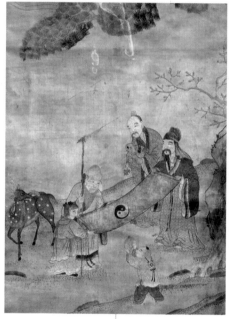

Above Three sages of Tai Chi surrounded by symbols of long life and immortality (tree, deer, peach). In the centre is Yin-Yang symbol.

The history of Tai Chi is a valuable aid to learning the art because it can help to give a greater depth of understanding to the art. As with any practice that can trace its history back through the centuries, there are many myths and legends surrounding Tai Chi.

One of the most interesting stories claims that Tai Chi was presented to a Taoist monk in the form of a dream by 'extraterrestrials', with instructions for the form to be transmitted to humankind. Many of the stories cite the Wudang Mountain in China as being the place of origin for Tai Chi. The art is indeed still practised there in modern times.

Many of the old Chinese texts take the Taoist priest Zhang Sangfeng, who lived in the fourteenth or fifteenth century, as the originator of Tai Chi. He is said to have witnessed a struggle between a snake and a crane, which gave him the inspiration for Tai Chi. The crane was trying to eat the snake, but could not pick it up to do so. The reason for this was that the snake stayed soft and supple whilst the crane was trying to devour it. The snake managed to wriggle out of the crane's clutches and was able to live another day.

A number of the stories about the origins of Tai Chi may owe as much to human imagination as to events that happened in reality. Like all of the Taoist stories, there is a grain of knowledge hidden within each of them.

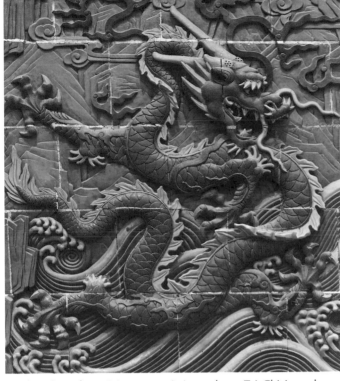

Left The dragon is a potent Yang symbol in Chinese mythology.

The idea of receiving transmissions about Tai Chi in a dream can be interpreted as using meditation to reach different levels of consciousness. Meditation can teach valuable lessons about oneself and Tai Chi. The story about the snake highlights the spiritual and meditative aspects of Tai Chi.

It may be that the legendary confrontation between the snake and the crane had very little to do with the actual origins of Tai Chi. In real life, some birds do manage to eat snakes without starving to death trying to catch them! The real point of the legend is to present the idea that softness is able to overcome rigidity. Although the snake may have had a few knocks and bruises from the escapade, it eventually escaped. The lithe movements of the snake enabled it to avoid the stabbing and grabbing of the bird's beak and claws.

This would be analogous to a person who, when threatened by a stronger force, does not respond with another show of force, but remains soft and relaxed and yields to the attack. The opponent will therefore have very little to attack and will leave themselves open to counterattack

11

Tai Chi Form

The style of Tai Chi explained in this book is the Yang style, as practised by the Yang family. There are one hundred and eight moves in the form. This makes learning the whole of the form a somewhat daunting task for the beginner.

I t is for that reason that the Simplified – or Basic – Form was invented. It has only twenty-four movements, yet contains all of the essences of Tai Chi. It is the Simplified Form that is shown in this book (see pages 98–157). One of the many advantages of learning the Yang style of Tai Chi is that it is the most common style in the world. This means that most cities or large towns will have a Tai Chi club that you can join, allowing you to train with more experienced Tai Chi people.

Energy

Intrinsic to Tai Chi is the idea of energy. When we talk about energy in this context, we are talking about the internal energy within the body – the energy that stops us from simply being a collection of chemical reactions and gives us life itself. The Chinese name for this energy is 'Chi'. The basic idea of 'Chi Energy' will be discussed on the following pages.

Yin and Yang

The ancient Chinese Yin/Yang symbol has become a fashionable piece of graphic artwork in recent years. Most people will be familiar with the circular shape that is black in one half and white in the other. From the many who have seen the symbol or even have it on their T-shirts, relatively few will be aware that the symbol is called the Tai Chi symbol or the symbol of the 'Supreme Ultimate'.

What the symbol illustrates is the interaction between the universal forces of Yin and Yang. This is the foundation upon which many philosophical concepts in Chinese culture are based. The idea of Yin and Yang is explained on the following page.

Yin and Yang

In Taoist cosmology, at the origin of the universe there was an empty state called Wu Chi – a nothingness symbolised by an empty circle. In the original void, forces started to attract and repel each other, until there were just two left: Yin and Yang.

The Yin and Yang forces coalesced together with such density that matter formed. It is from this concentration of Yin and Yang forces into matter that the 'Ten Thousand Things' of the physical universe were born. The phrase 'Ten Thousand Things' is not a literal phrase but is simply a large number used to represent all the individual items in the universe.

The implication of this is that everything around us consists of Yin and Yang forces and contained within them are the origins of the universe. This worldview is not entirely at odds with the findings of modern physics. The theory that energy and matter are the same is also stated in Einstein's famous equation: $E = MC^2$ (where E = energy, M = mass (or matter) and C = speed of light).

Above The Yin and Yang symbol represents the two complementary forces that make up our universe.

Yin and Yang in Tai Chi

The concept of Yin and Yang forms the philosophical framework upon which the art of Tai Chi was founded. The starting posture of the Tai Chi Form is called the Wu Chi posture and symbolises nothingness, or emptiness. As the arms begin to lift for the first movement, the internal forces of Yin and Yang are starting to define themselves. When The Form starts to move, we are constantly using contraction and expansion (Yin and Yang). The movement of The Form through the Yin and Yang energies is a microcosm of the Ten Thousand Things. At the end of the form, all energy returns to where it started from – the Wu Chi posture.

13

Energy Chi

The concept of Chi (or Qi) is central to Tai Chi and other healing and martial arts throughout the world. Chi has been a source of debate for centuries and will most probably stay that way for centuries yet to come.

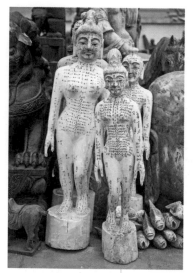

Above Chinese acupuncture statues. Chi flows through the body along the meridians. Blockages in the Chi can be treated with acupuncture.

One of the major causes for debate is that Chi is the nonphysical, or etheric, part of a person. Some very learned individuals therefore dismiss the concept, as the etheric body is invisible to the untrained eye so they think that it cannot exist.

The fundamental view of the human body, as outlined by Chinese medicine, states that the organisation of the energetic part of the human body precedes the organisation of the physical part of the human body. This means it is the movement of Chi throughout the body that brings about all thoughts, emotions and physical movements of the human body.

Another implication is that if one person can alter his or her own energetic body – or that of someone else – then it is also possible to alter the state of mind or body. Healers and martial artists who use Chi as a part of their treatments and processes will therefore be doing exactly that.

One of the aims of Tai Chi practice is to refine our Chi. By refining the energetic body, refinements will also be made to our body, mind and spirit. In this way we have the potential to heal ourselves through practising Tai Chi.

There are different manifestations of Chi. An inanimate object has Chi, but has no life. This would mean that it has no 'Jing'. Jing is the manifestation of Chi that allows life to be present within a thing. A good example would be that a building would have its own Chi but no Jing.

All living things are said to have Jing. If a living thing has another quality of Chi called 'Shen', then it will have the capability of self-reflection. Traditional Chinese medicine believes that human beings are the only creatures capable of Shen. Furthermore, those people with a great amount of Shen will be capable of the greatest self-reflection. According to this reasoning, Buddha would have possessed large amounts of Shen.

There are three sources of Chi available to us. These are the Chi that we are born with, the Chi that we get from our food, and the Chi that we get through breathing. If we stop getting enough of either food Chi or air Chi, we become ill (naturally, we cannot alter the Chi we are born with). When practising Tai Chi, the breathing always comes from the stomach. The reason for this is that our reservoir of Chi is situated in the stomach. By breathing Chi into the stomach, we top up our Chi reserves and, in doing so, increase our vital energy.

Below Traditional Chinese medical practitioners re-establish the balance of Yin and Yang in the body by manipulating Chi through acupuncture, herbal medicine and Chi Kung.

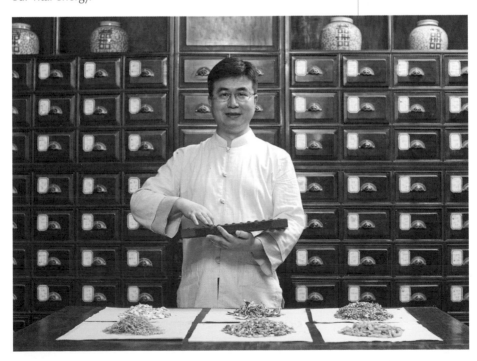

How to use this Book

At the core of this book, The Form offers a twenty-four-step program of Yang-style Tai Chi. The chapters leading up to it can be seen as a means of preparation for performing it. They include an introduction to the basics of Tai Chi, a series of warm-up exercises, and two series of Chi Kung exercises. The chapters that follow The Form discuss applications of Tai Chi in greater detail.

A sequence transition follows each exercise and explains how to move seamlessly from one exercise to the next without stopping the flow of movement.

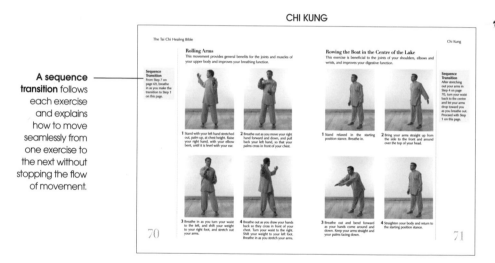

Chi Kung

Two chapters on the art of Chi Kung introduce beginners to the idea of Chi – the flow of energy throughout the body. The sequences demonstrated are considerably shorter than those of The Form. As such, they allow the beginner to practise calm, fluid movements as he or she progresses from one exercise to the next. Above all they teach the beginner the importance of being able to focus the mind, a crucial element of the art of Tai Chi. As the movement progresses from one exercise to the next, there is advice on making the 'sequence transition' as fluid as possible.

THE FORM

The Tai Chi Healing Bible The Form

Step 7: Grasp the Bird's Tail – Left Style

Points to Remember
• In step 55 of the Bird's Tail, your feet and waist make the same left bow stance as in Part Wild Horse Mane (see page 102) but your left arm is bent across your chest and not raised.

49 Bring your left hand level with your ear and turn to the right. Push your left hand forward.

50 As your hands move, raise your right foot and step back as before, this time shifting your weight to the right foot.

52 Turn to the right. Move your right hand up and to the side, to shoulder height, palm facing up, while your left hand is palm down. Look at your left hand.

53 Make a hold-ball in front of your right side, with your right hand on top. Shift your weight onto your right foot, draw your left foot, on its toes, next to your right foot.

Points to Remember
• You step back four times: with your left foot, right foot, and left and right again.
• When stepping back, place your toes down first and then set the entire foot on the floor.
• Turn your front stra ightens ely with the body turn, pivoting on your toes, until the foot comes in line with your body.
• Move your left leg slightly toward the left – or right leg slightly toward the right, as the case may be – when taking a step backward, being careful not to let the feet land in a straight line.

51 Bring your left hand level with your ear and turn to the right. Push your left hand forward.

54 Turn your body slightly to the left, raise your left foot and step forward.

55 Turn a little more to the left, and complete the left bow stance. Push out your left forearm, palm in. Drop your right hand by your right hip, palm down.

116 117

Points to **Remember** list suggestions for improving a stance or a transition into the next move, and offer hints and tips for the right posture to adapt as you perform a given exercise.

The Form

This chapter presents the one hundred and fifty-nine steps that make up The Form, broken down into twenty-nine exercises. Like the Chi Kung exercises, the intention here is to practise the steps in order to perform the entire sequence without interruption. With practice, an individual should be able to maintain the same speed of movement throughout, while focusing on the flow of Chi through his or her body. Throughout the chapter are 'points to remember', which enable beginners of The Form to perfect their movements through slight adjustments to posture. The following chapter, The Form at a Glance, offers nine steps per page, allowing practitioners who have mastered The Form to progress with even greater speed and fluidity.

Practical Considerations

• Decide on a fixed time of day for your practice – any time during the day.
• Morning practice of Chi Kung (see pages 62–85) and The Form (see pages 98–157) will energise you for the rest of the day, while performing meditation exercises in the evening will help you unwind.
• If practising indoors, choose a quiet, well-ventilated room.
• Practise outdoors whenever you can.
• Aim to practise for a minimum of 20 to 30 minutes daily.
• Wear loose clothes that do not constrict your waist or chest, nor impede the free movement of your limbs.
• Always wear footwear, especially if practising outdoors – comfortable flat-soled slippers that allow you to feel the ground.

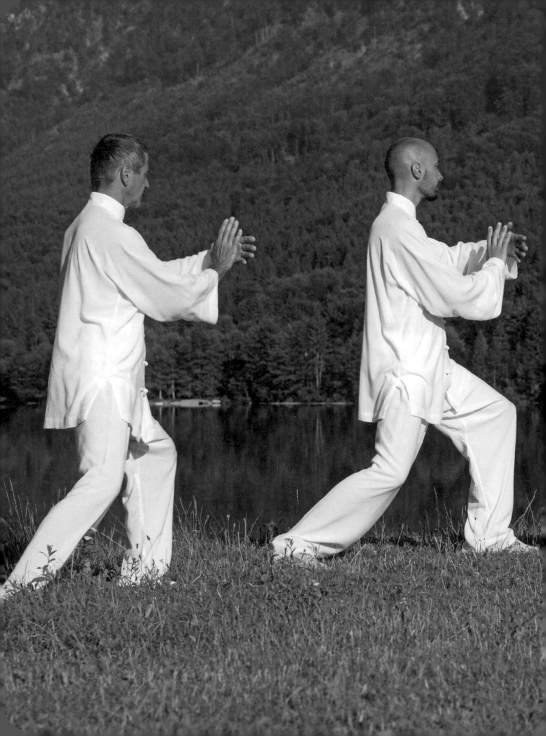

Tai Chi Basics

In order to practise Tai Chi successfully, it is first necessary to master a handful of basic techniques. These include the Ten Essences of Tai Chi, the Tai Chi Stances, and the Tai Chi Hand Positions.

The Ten Essences of Tai Chi

The Ten Essences of Tai Chi were developed by Yang Cheng Fu to help his students understand the movements of The Form. Yang Cheng Fu was living in China between 1883 and 1936. He adapted the Yang-style Tai Chi Form to the series of movements we know today.

Opposite A bad posture will need correcting before correct Tai Chi can be practised.

The ten essences are:

1. Lift the head to raise the spirit
2. Lower the shoulders to sink the elbows
3. Curve the back and soften the chest
4. Loosen the waist
5. Be aware of weight distribution
6. Coordinate the top half of the body with the bottom half of the body
7. Continuity in movement
8. Unite the mind (intent) with the body (frame)
9. Use mind and not force
10. Seek stillness within motion and motion within stillness

The Ten Essences of Tai Chi have become an invaluable learning aid to many exponents of the art. When fully understood, the ten essences define a type of body structure rather than trying to dictate actual moves. The ten essences can therefore be valuable knowledge to any martial arts student (no matter what style), and even to dance students, since the principles are pretty much the same. When watching a well-trained dancer, one will usually be able to see the ten essences in place.

The ten essences can therefore be regarded as the building blocks of Tai Chi Chuan. If any one of these essences is not in place, the student will have great difficulty attaining anything close to a high skill level in the art.

A New Order

When Yang Cheng Fu developed the Ten Essences of Tai Chi, they were presented in no particular order. More recently, however, Christopher Pei, a modern Tai Chi master of great reputation, has revisited the ten essences. He has shown that they can be rearranged into a chronological order of skill level.

This means that it is helpful to work on the essences in the order in which they follow (see opposite page). A student's time is therefore better spent practising the first essences in the form and gradually moving on to the later ones, than working on the later essences first. And so it follows that one may be able to assess a Tai Chi practitioner's skill level in the art by observing which of the ten essences are in place.

The Physical Essences

The first five of the ten essences are physical essences, which establish the right conditions in the body for the correct practice of Tai Chi Chuan. Without the physical conditions that are fulfilled by the first five of the ten essences, it is not possible to successfully develop the last five of the ten essences.

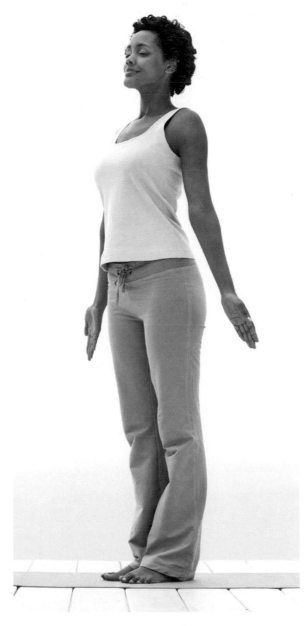

This would be similar to an architect trying to build a great building but having weak foundations. Sooner or later the building will topple, and will have to be rebuilt. It would have been better in the long run to have spent more time on the foundations. The architect could have then built higher without finishing with a pile of rubble. If the architect still wants to create his masterpiece, he will do no better unless he alters the foundations, so effectively he will have to start again. To avoid having to start again with Tai Chi, get the ten essences correct in the first place and you will be able to build as high as you want.

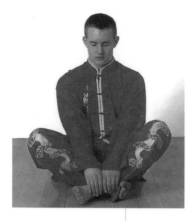

Above Achieving harmony between the body and mind is at the heart of the Ten Essences of Tai Chi.

Mind, Body, Spirit

The first of the five physical essences starts at the head. The fifth finishes at the feet. It is therefore possible, once these essences have been understood, to use them as a physical checklist at any point in The Form to check posture.

Once the physical requirements of the first five essences are in place, work will automatically begin on essences six to ten. The key word to these essences is coordination. When we study Tai

Right The ten essences can help correct a too-tense body.

Far Right It may take time to achieve the correct stance, but it is worth persevering.

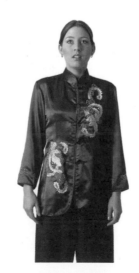

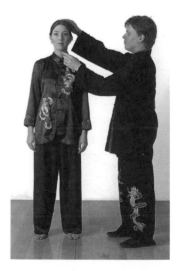

Chi Chuan, one of our aims can be coordination, or strengthening the links between mind, body and spirit.

This is indeed a lofty sounding goal, and needs explanation to become a practical piece of knowledge rather than yet more esoteric rhetoric.

When we are working on essences six and seven, we are mostly working with the coordination of the upper and lower body. On eight and nine, we are uniting mind and body. By the time we reach the last essence, number ten, we are working mostly with spirit.

The Ten Essences of Tai Chi effectively form a 'map' that will help you to chart the previously unknown country of body, mind and spirit. By working patiently and methodically, you will gain an understanding of the last essences.

This then begs the question of what happens after the tenth essence. Will you know everything about Tai Chi? The answer to this question can actually be found in the first essence, which refers to spirit.

Originally you will have simply lifted the head. At first it will be difficult enough just to maintain this throughout The Form. After working through the essences, you will have made changes to your body, energy and understanding of the basics. You should now understand 'Lift the Head to Raise the Spirit' in a completely different way from when you started. The task now is to apply that new understanding to the Tai Chi Form.

This is how the ten essences can be used as a tool for the continuous development of your Tai Chi Chuan.

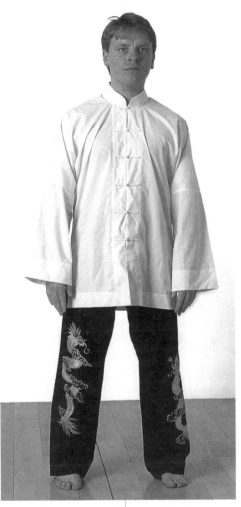

Above The ten essences coordinate the body's positioning and energies.

23

The First Essence

Next time you are in a waiting room or other busy place, take a look at the people around you. You will probably see that many people are wandering around with their heads bowed, looking at either the floor or their shoes. The reasons for this can be varied; they could be ill, tired or sad.

Lift the head to raise the spirit

To practise the first essence, stand straight and hold the neck and head upright, but relaxed. Imagine the mind concentrated together at the top of the head. This should also be relaxed, otherwise the flow of Chi will be interrupted.

If your head is bowed, then your spirit cannot be high. Simply by straightening your back and lifting your head, the spirit will lift. A person who feels that they have 'the weight of the world on their shoulders' will not have good spirit. Next time you are feeling a bit like this, consider how you are holding your body and straighten up a bit to lift the spirit. In this way you are teaching yourself to 'walk tall'.

From a martial artist's point of view, this is probably the most important of all the essences. The first thing that two competitors will do is look at each other. Imagine that one competitor has his head raised and is looking relaxed. Then imagine that the opponent only half looks up, and half looks downward. The body language has already told you where to place your bets.

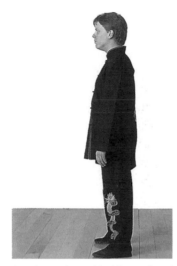

Stand straight and hold your head and neck upright, but relaxed.

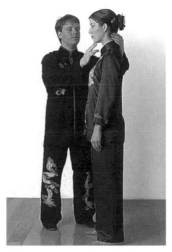

Lifting your head will lift your spirits.

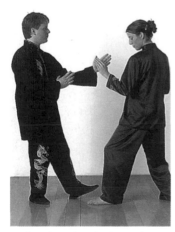

With the head bowed, an opponent looks defeated from the beginning.

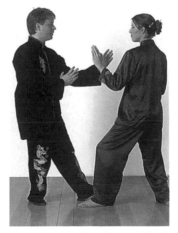

Now with the head raised, both opponents are evenly matched.

25

The Second Essence

In Tai Chi, there will always be a pairing of Yin and Yang. It follows that if the head is raised, then something must be lowered. If the shoulders are not lowered, energy becomes trapped high up on the body and is useless.

Lower the shoulders to sink the elbows

P rove this to yourself by standing up and lifting your shoulders as high as you can for a couple of minutes. Try to lift your shoulders so high that they are touching your ears.

Then suddenly release them, and feel the relief. After a while it becomes a real physical strain to keep your shoulders high. On a smaller scale, even if your shoulders are only slightly raised, precious energy is simply being wasted.

For the martial artist, the basic mechanics illustrate the point. If the shoulders are high, the centre of gravity will be raised. For maximum stability in any structure, the centre of gravity should be low. It therefore makes sense that the person with the lower centre of gravity has a lower possibility of being knocked over.

A good tip for this is to try to keep the elbows pointing down to the floor. If the elbows are pointing down, then the shoulders will be down, too.

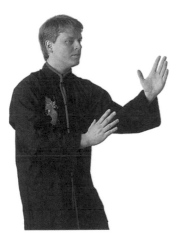

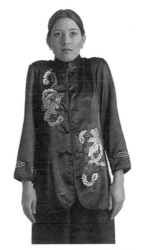

Here the shoulders are lowered and the elbows dipped.

Holding your shoulders high for any length of time is a great strain.

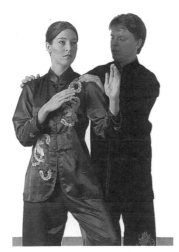

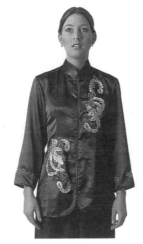

It will take effort to keep the shoulders relaxed.

Once you can keep your shoulders lowered, you will have enhanced your energy.

The Third Essence

Stand to attention! Chin up! Shoulders back! Feet together! This has become a part of the physical conditioning of our culture. Whether in the services, at school, or simply picking the idea up from the television, many people have similar body dynamics to this.

Soften the chest and curve the back

The opposite end of this scale is a slumped posture that pushes the abdomen forward, which affects the working of the internal organs.

Instead of pulling the shoulders back, fold them forward gently. Make sure that your back is straight, your head up, and your shoulders down (from essences one and two, pages 24 and 26). Repeat the mental checks that you did while standing in the 'Attention!' posture.

You may now find that your breathing can become softer and that your abdomen will start to move with your breathing. The reason for this is that the energy meridian for the lungs has become softer, thus allowing your breathing to become deeper. The important part of this meridian is at its end. This point lies just below your shoulders and needs to be relaxed to allow your breathing to relax.

When your breathing becomes relaxed, your body can become relaxed, too. Your skeleton itself will have less pressure on it from bad body posture, and your internal organs will also become less restricted as a result of this.

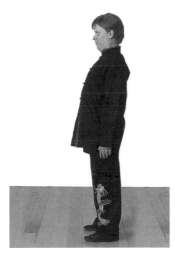

Many people make the mistake of standing to attention, puffing their chests out.

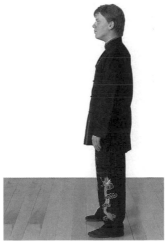

A relaxed posture with back straight is correct.

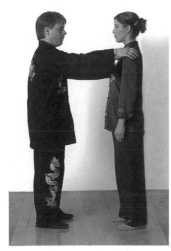

You may need help to achieve this posture.

29

The Fourth Essence

When the physical requirements of the first three essences have been attained, your body will have started to relax and become softer. This allows your breathing to sink to the Tan Tien.

Loosen the waist

The Tan Tien is a very important point within the Tai Chi system, as it is with other martial and healing arts. It is an invisible energy centre that is positioned just below the navel. Other names for it are the 'sea of Ki' or centre of the 'Hara'. These are both Japanese phrases for the same thing.

The important point is that the Tan Tien radiates energy out to the rest of the body. It can be felt and its effects observed, but it is not a physical entity that can be seen with normal vision.

When most people first see Tai Chi being performed, they notice the movement of the arms and legs. Indeed many Tai Chi practitioners only move the limbs. For Tai Chi to be done properly, the movement should come from the Tan Tien. Movement of the arms and legs within Tai Chi should be like ripples coming from the Tan Tien.

A useful piece of advice here is that, when learning a new move in the Tai Chi (or re-learning an old one), do not be confused by the hands and feet. Try to see the body as a unified entity, with the centre of movement being the waist. Try to work out how to move the waist so that the desired movement happens. When Tai Chi moves are incorrectly executed, it is usually the waist that is wrong. You will save a great deal of time if you address your movement from the waist as soon as possible, rather than trying to work out where your hands and feet should be. The movement will then be more grounded and intuitive.

If your breathing sinks into the Tan Tien by using the first three essences, then the Tan Tien will become stronger. This will allow the movements to be issued from your waist, or the Tan Tien. For this to happen, your waist must be free to move. If your waist will not allow this freedom of movement, the ripples on our pond of energy will be more like throwing a pebble into mud: No energy will be allowed to travel outward.

The first essences effectively set up the conditions for the upper body. You have now moved down to the waist and are setting up conditions for the lower body. One thing that should have remained with you throughout is the idea of letting go of tension. Starting with the upper body, this release of tension continues at the waist.

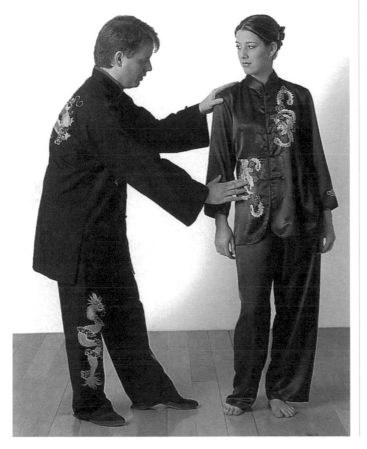

Left Loosening the waist completes the correct posture procedure for the upper body.

31

The Fifth Essence

To gain a feeling of what essence five is teaching, stand for a while in a natural posture. At this moment you are not particularly concerned about what the stance is, you are simply looking at the feelings within the stance.

Be aware of weight distribution

S ettle into the stance, and then start to go through the essences that you have learnt so far. Lift up your head, let your shoulders drop down, and allow your breathing to soften. Relax your waist, keep your spine straight, and do not allow your bottom to poke out. Let your breathing become soft, so that when you breathe in, your abdomen comes out and when you breathe out, your abdomen comes in. Now check your knees and ankles. They should be relaxed. Never allow your knee joints to lock up. Make sure that the joints are relaxed by bending them slightly. Do not forget that your back has to be straight, even if your knees are bent, so do not tip your body forward or backward.

Now feel the weight in your feet. Your weight distribution should be divided equally between each foot. Try playing with your weight distribution. Push the heel of your left foot into the floor gradually, so that the distribution changes from fifty-fifty to sixty-forty, then from sixty-forty to seventy-thirty and so on until all your weight is on your left leg. Try doing this exercise several times until you can change the weight distribution from foot to foot without altering the alignment of your body. You may find that this exercise requires more effort than you anticipated. The reason for this is that altering the weight in the legs as you have just done is automatically altering the feeling of 'rooting'.

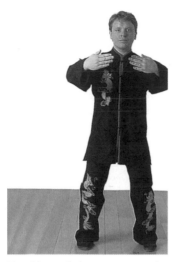

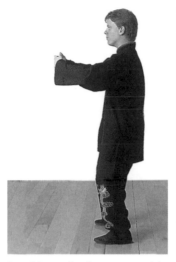

To achieve a balance, you must be aware of the weight in your feet.

Practising adjusting your weight distribution is vital for correct Tai Chi movements.

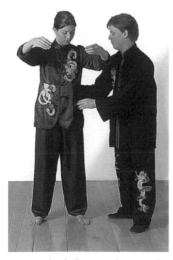

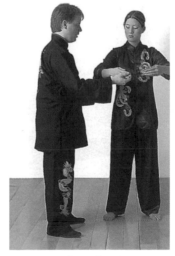

Getting the balance right can take time and effort.

You may well need an instructor's help before mastering this technique.

33

The Sixth Essence

Imagine an army going into battle. This army has a problem at the moment. The trouble is that half the soldiers are at home watching the television. The remaining soldiers on the front line will not be as effective, because they have not managed to mobilise all their forces.

Coordinate the top half of the body with the bottom

Mobilisation of the whole of the forces within the body is one of the fundamental requirements of Tai Chi. For example, during a push, the beginner will usually perform the push with the top half of the body only. This will mean that the bottom half of the body (where the strongest muscles are) is not being used in the push.

The more experienced Tai Chi student, who can use the legs for the push, as well as the arms, will have a stronger technique. The reason for this is that the second student has managed to use the whole of the body, rather than just the top half. This is why you must pay attention to the coordination of the upper and lower halves of your body.

This is quite easy to observe. When a move is coming forward, your knee should stop moving at the same time as your elbow. If one part of your body finishes before the other part, the coordination of your upper and lower body is at fault.

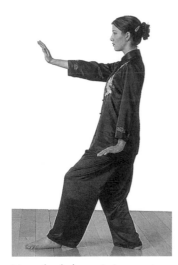

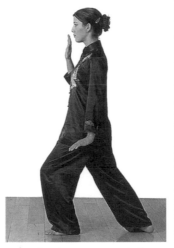

Here the balance is incorrect, as the back leg is bent.

Again this shows incorrect balance, as the arms have not gone forward to balance the legs.

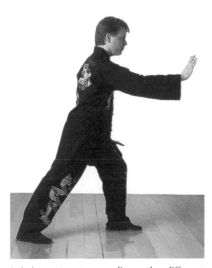

It is important to coordinate the different parts of the body. Here the legs and arms are balanced.

The Seventh Essence

Think back to the army that we spoke of during the last essence. This time the soldiers are more focused. They are marching in the morning this time, so there is nothing to distract them from their task. Unfortunately, some of the soldiers stayed up rather late and are suffering from tiredness.

Continuity in movement

This tiredness gradually becomes all they can think about, so some of the soldiers stop for a short break, promising that they will catch up soon. This would obviously be a hazardous situation. There is nothing to gain from mobilising the whole army if they are not coordinated. The group of soldiers needs to be constantly in motion to be effective, otherwise there will still only be half of the army meeting any attack.

This same logic applies to Tai Chi. Once the body starts to move, it should stay moving. Different parts of the body will move at different speeds, but at no time should any part of the body stop so that another part can catch up.

This also shows how closely essences six and seven are linked. If the movement is being generated from the waist, and the top and bottom halves of the body are coordinated, the movement will be continuous. If the legs are moving before the arms, or vice versa, one part of the body will have to stop so that the other can catch up, and the movement will not be continuous.

Coordinated movement allows the form to become soft and continuous and sets up the pre-requisites for energy flow.

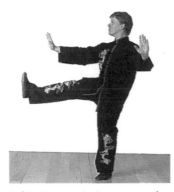

Achieving continuity means that the various parts of the body move in harmony.

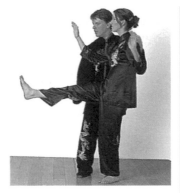

Here the movement has not been continuous, as the leg has not moved at the same time as the torso.

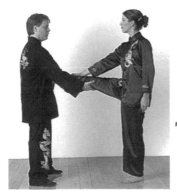

You will probably need help to coordinate your movements correctly.

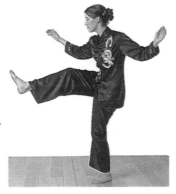

Eventually you will find that flowing movement comes naturally.

The Eighth Essence

Let us go back to see how our soldiers are faring. They are looking very much improved. They are all working together and the whole army looks and feels better. The men no longer feel like a collection of parts, but are a coordinated group instead.

Unite mind and body

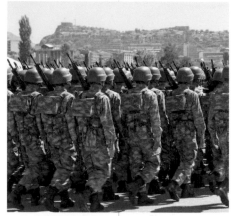

Above An army needs to have a balance between the physical unity of the soldiers, and their awareness and readiness for battle.

The truth, however, is slightly different. They look good and feel good, but if they were to face another army they would be in trouble. The reason for this is that while being excellent at marching, they have little or no idea of what to do when they meet the enemy.

This would be similar to the Tai Chi student who can exercise the moves, but has no true understanding of them, or what they are used for. Tai Chi was invented and evolved as a martial art. If the Tai Chi student understands the martial application of the moves, he or she can use the intent of the mind to increase the flow of Chi.

Without the intent, the moves become little more than waving the arms and legs. This may be enough for a simple keep-fit exercise, but if you want all the benefits that Tai Chi has to offer, you must use the mind and the intent.

Only when you can use intent properly will your energy flow be at its strongest and you will achieve the best possible healing effect on your body.

The Ninth Essence

Tai Chi is classified by many as a 'soft' or 'internal' martial art. The meaning of 'soft' in this context relates to how you hold your muscles. With 'internal' martial arts, power doesn't come from strength alone.

Use mind not force

This is one feature of Tai Chi that is frequently not understood. Many Tai Chi students learn how to be soft, but they do not actually generate any power.

The reason that little or no power has been generated is that they have not understood the use of mind or 'intent'. Energy cannot flow without intent, and without intent, the Tai Chi will not be complete.

The reason that we have to be soft is to allow our energy meridians to become relaxed. Energy flows through the body via a system of channels or 'meridians'. Energy cannot flow powerfully without intent, thus without intent your Tai Chi will not be complete.

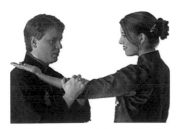

Unlike other martial arts, Tai Chi does not rely on muscular strength.

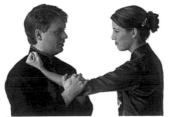

Rather, Tai Chi uses the flow of energy to create 'intent' which increases power.

39

The Tenth Essence

When one progresses into these realms of the mind and body, words cannot convey the whole of our experience (remember our original definition of Tai Chi). The tenth essence involves quite a high level of meditation.

Seek stillness within motion and motion within stillness

An analogy for the tenth essence comes from a film in which a basketball team has trouble shooting. The coach tells them that whenever they have possession of the ball they need to be able to stop, take a breath and shoot. Basketball is a fast game and the coach is asking her players to find stillness within motion, which may seem impossible, yet it is not. When stillness within motion is found, the inner body has the feeling of extension and creation of energy. This is how you will find motion within stillness and be able to complete the tenth essence.

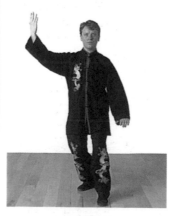

Achieving stillness is an important part of Tai Chi practice.

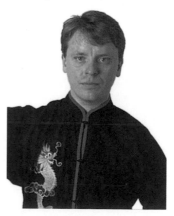

Combining motion and stillness is the key to successfully completing the ten essences.

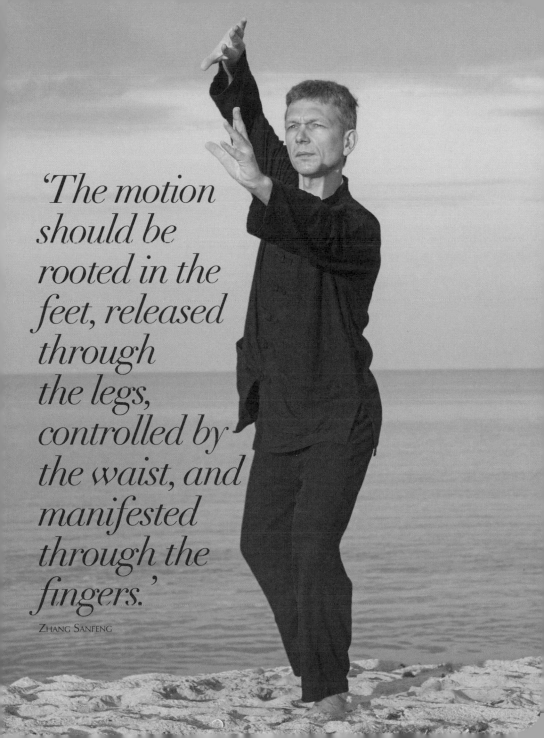

'The motion should be rooted in the feet, released through the legs, controlled by the waist, and manifested through the fingers.'

ZHANG SANFENG

Tai Chi Stances

In Yang-style Tai Chi there are only four stances. If you find that you are standing in any other stance during the form, then it is wrong and needs correcting. It is therefore essential to gain a good understanding of the postures.

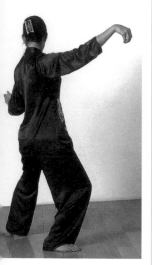

Above Drop Stance

Parallel Stance

Used in the opening form, closing form and Wave Hands like Clouds. This is the only stance during the whole of the form where the weight is equal on both legs. This only occurs during the opening and commencing forms. The weight is actually shifting during Wave Hands like Clouds, but the posture remains the same.

Bow Stance

Used in Part Wild Horse Mane on Both Sides, Brush Knee and Twist Step, Grasp the Bird's Tail, Single Whip, Fair Lady Works Shuttles, Fan Penetrates Back, Parry and Punch, and Withdraw and Push.

The weight is approximately 70 percent on the front leg and 30 percent on the back leg. There are two variations of the Bow Stance. One is where the torso of the body and the back leg are straight, and the other is where the torso is vertical.

Empty Stance

Used in White Crane Spreads its Wings, Hand Strums the Lute, Step Back to Drive Monkey Away, High Pat on Horse, Kicks, Squat Down and Stand on One Leg and Needle at Sea Bottom. The Empty Stance is regarded by many as the most difficult. This is because all your weight is supported entirely on your back leg.

Drop Stance

Used only with Squat Down and Stand on One Leg, the Drop Stance is very similar to the Bow Stance, except that your weight is on your back leg and your torso has dropped lower.

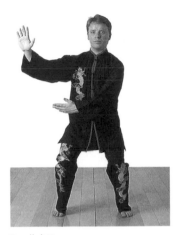

Parallel Stance

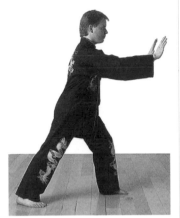

Bow Stance

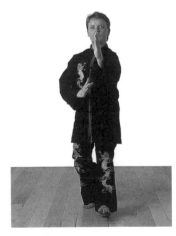

Empty Stance

Tai Chi Hand Positions

A simple and easy way for the beginner to judge the skill level of a person more experienced in Tai Chi is to look at the person's hands when they are practising. The reason for this is not that the hand movements are excessively complicated, but the opposite: the shapes of the hands in Tai Chi are deceptively simple.

There are three shapes for the hands in the Simplified Tai Chi Form: the open hand, the fist, and the 'tiger's mouth'. If you have managed to achieve the skill level where you do not need to 'try' to remember The Form, then you will be able to give more of your attention to the hands.

Open Hand (Tai Chi Palm)

A common mistake is to hold your hands limp. This stops energy travelling to your fingertips, making them appear lifeless. Limpness in the hand will also deny any understanding of martial applications, and therefore the intent is not exercised. The correct way to hold the hand for the Tai Chi Palm is somewhere in between a limp and a tight hand. The fingers should be extended, but also relaxed. The thumb is relaxed and quite close to the hand. This allows proper circulation of blood and energy so the hands feel more alive.

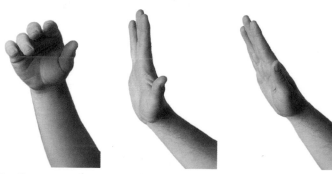

Too limp   Too tight   Extended but relaxed

Tai Chi Fist

Fists are used quite frequently toward the latter end of The Form. The fist in Tai Chi is similar to the fist used in many other martial arts, except that it is relaxed. If the fist becomes too tense, it will need correcting.

To make the Tai Chi fist, start by making the Tai Chi palm. Now roll the fingers toward the hand, so that they touch the palm. Finish the fist by bringing the thumb down over the first two fingers.

A common mistake is to bend the wrist when making a fist. The energy to the fist should come in a straight line from the elbow. If you bend your wrist, you will simply not be able to transmit any appreciable power through the fist. Also, if you prefer to think in martial arts terms, if you were to hit anything with a fist that was bent, you would hurt your wrist.

Another common mistake is to make a 'hollow' fist. This is again incorrect for the style of Tai Chi studied here.

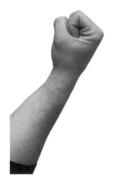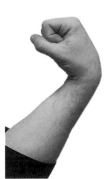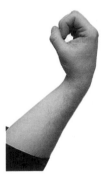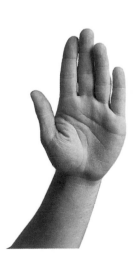

Correct fist   Incorrect: bent wrist   Incorrect: hollow fist

Tiger's Mouth

After learning the Tai Chi palm, the 'tiger's mouth' is easy. To make the shape for tiger's mouth, simply make the Tai Chi palm and move the thumb outward. Keep the hand relaxed but extended as before. This hand shape only occurs in Hand Strums the Lute.

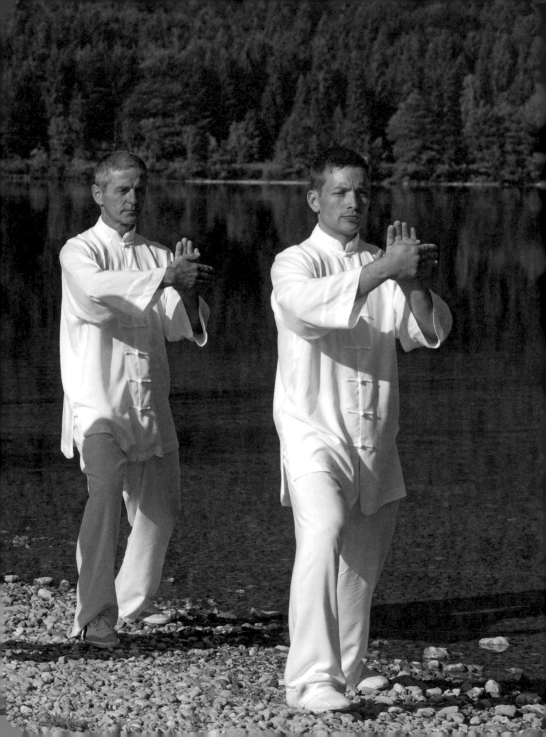

Warming Up

As with all forms of martial arts, it is essential to perform some warm-up exercises before practising Tai Chi. An essential part of this is keeping the mind focused on the fluidity of your movements.

Body in Motion

From the macrocosm of the planet's orbit around the Sun to the microcosm of the electron's path around the nucleus of an atom, nature moves in spirals. So, in Tai Chi, which seeks to follow the laws of natural motion, you will find no straight lines. When you perform the Tai Chi Form and Chi Kung exercises, your posture and movements should immediately suggest roundness: Your chest is sunken, not puffed out; your arms and legs are relaxed and bent, never straight and stiff; your movements have the fluidity and smoothness of water, never hard or jerking.

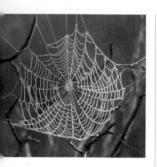

S piralling arms is a preparatory exercise that allows you to discover and explore the basic principles of Tai Chi motion and, as your skill increases, to monitor your progress. Do not worry if, in the beginning, your movements lack coordination or do not exactly match the illustrations. It is more important that you find your body's centre of gravity, and, keeping your mind fixed there, work to develop a smooth, continuous motion with which you feel completely comfortable. With practice, spiralling arms will become automatic; so, to ensure that your mind does not wander, always keep it focused on the movement.

'In motion all parts of the body must be light, nimble, and strung together.'

ZHANG SANFENG

Spiralling Arms

Stand with one foot in front of, and at right angles to, the other.

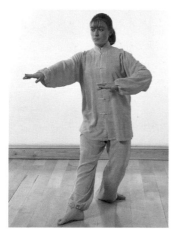

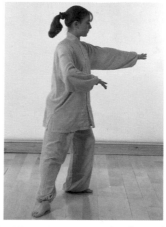

1 Gently rock backward and forward. Raise your arms to waist height, shoulders relaxed, and make circles with your hands, palms facing down.

2 Without interrupting the flow of the movement, turn your waist in time to the spiralling of your arms and the shifting of your weight.

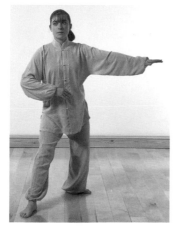

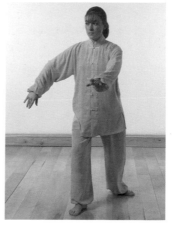

3 Feel the connection between your feet, waist and shoulders in one seamless movement. Make sure you maintain a constant speed.

4 Identify any stiffness or weakness in your body. These areas will require special attention during your further study of Tai Chi.

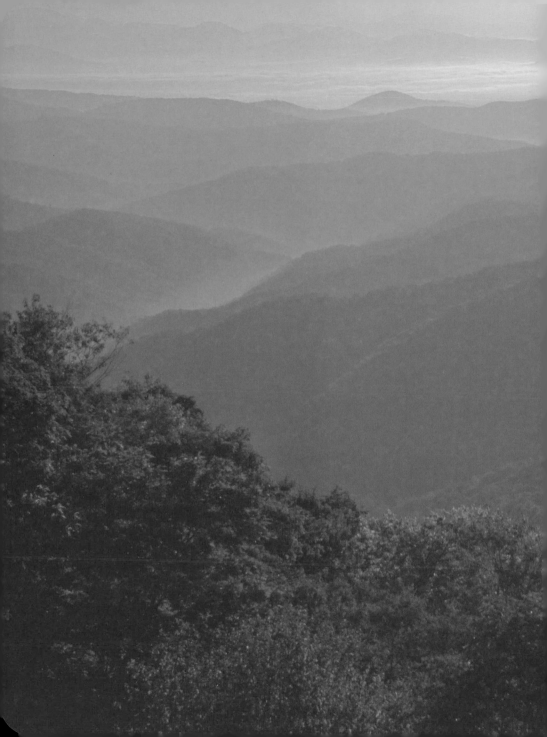

'In the morning of your practice, your muscles and joints are stiff and your bones are hollow. At noontime, the Chi flows freely into your Tan Tien; and in the evening of your practice the Chi congeals in your marrow, turning it to steel.'

Opening the Energy Gates

As you begin your practice of Tai Chi, you will notice that it shares many features familiar to you from other forms of exercise: wearing specialist clothing and shoes, for example, or going to a room or area set aside for practice, and performing preparatory warm-up exercises.

I n Tai Chi, whose aim is to bring the mental and physical aspects of movement into complete harmony, a period of preparation to relax and prepare the mind and body is also necessary, and as your practice progresses, you may wish to perform meditation and breathing exercises before you begin your daily round of exercises. The following movements are designed to stretch and mobilise your joints and major muscle groups. For your Tai Chi practice, they also serve to clear any blockages in your Chi and stimulate its flow throughout your body.

Rotating the Wrists

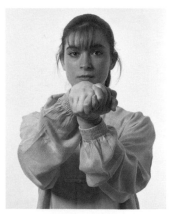 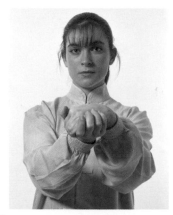

1 Keeping your shoulders and elbows relaxed, clasp your hands together in front of you, and make a figure of eight in one direction.

2 Repeat the movement in the opposite direction. Don't let tension build up in the muscles of your neck and upper back.

Rotating the Elbows

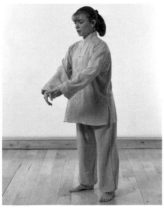

1 Stand with your feet shoulder-width apart and start to raise your arms in front of you.

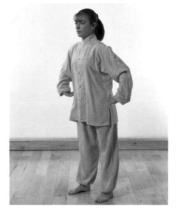

2 Keeping your shoulders and upper back relaxed, make circles with your forearms, rotating from your elbows.

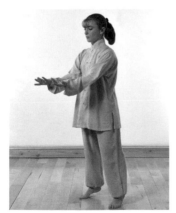

3 As you rotate your forearms, rise onto the balls of your feet.

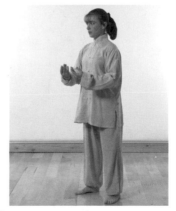

4 Slowly raise and lower your body, keeping in time with the movement of your arms.

53

Rotating the Shoulders

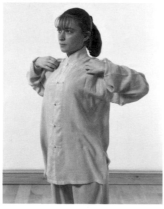 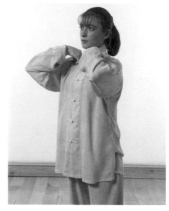

1 With your hands resting loosely on your shoulders, make circles with your elbows.

2 Move in a forward direction, and then a backward direction.

Rotating the Hips

Rotating the Knees

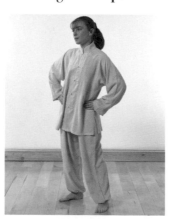 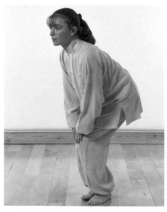

Stand with your legs shoulder-width apart. Put your hands on your hips, and rotate your body clockwise and counterclockwise for two full turns.

Stand with your feet together, knees bent. Hold your knees as you rotate them one way and then the other.

Pulling Back the Arms

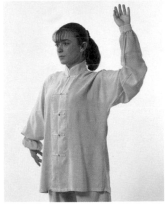

1 Slowly raise one arm while lowering the other.

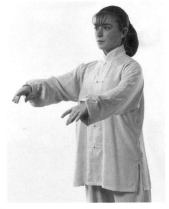

2 Repeat the movement twice.

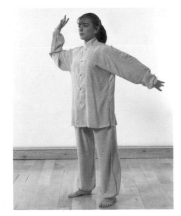

3 Reverse the positions of your arms.

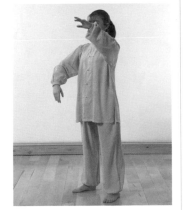

4 Repeat the movement twice.

'Remember when moving there is no place that does not move.'

Wu Yuxiang

Wild Goose Reaches for the Sky

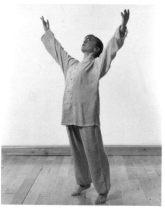 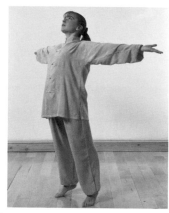

1 Stand with your feet shoulder-width apart, arms hanging loosely at your sides. Breathe in, raise and open your arms toward the sky, and rise to the balls of your feet.

2 Hold the position momentarily, then breathe out as you lower your arms and body.

Turning Waist to Swing Arms

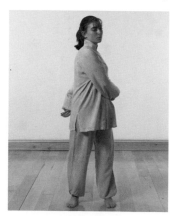

Turn your waist from left to right, shifting your weight from one foot to the other, as your arms swing freely.

Turning Step to Swing Arms

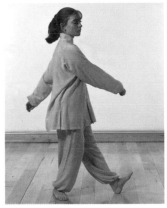 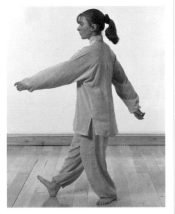

1 As you swing, raise one foot onto its heel.

2 Turn the foot out as the opposing arm swings forward.

Turning Waist to Pat the Back

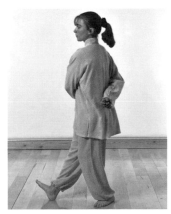 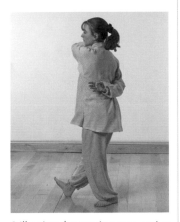

3 Your foot should be in position before your waist begins to turn.

Still using the turning step, swing your hands over your shoulders and pat yourself lightly. Do not force a stretch in this movement, but go only as far as the swing naturally takes your hand.

57

Turning Step with Walking Swing

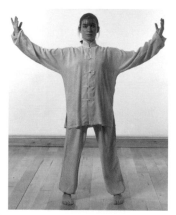

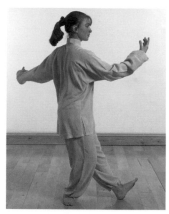

1 Using the same turning step technique for your feet as in the previous exercises, swing the arms up to shoulder height.

2 Swing them down in opposite directions, making two smooth, sweeping arcs.

Rotating your Ankles

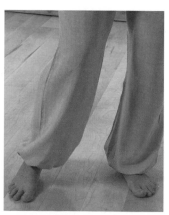

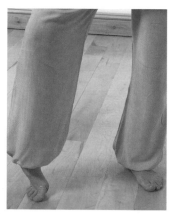

1 Resting your weight on your left foot, rotate your right ankle in a clockwise direction.

2 Rotate the same ankle in a counter-clockwise direction. Repeat with your weight on your right foot.

Hamstring Stretch

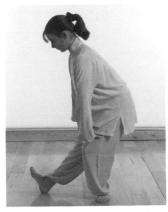

Stand with legs apart and take a step forward, to stand on your right heel. Hands on knees, bend forward from the waist. Repeat with the left foot.

Raised Rear- and Inner-thigh Stretch

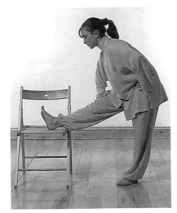

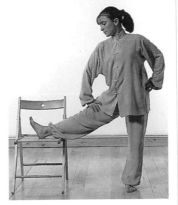

1 Rest your foot on a raised surface, such as a chair,. Keeping your back leg straight and your foot flat on the floor, bend forward to stretch your hamstring.

2 Straighten your body, turn to the front, and bend sideways to stretch the inner thigh. Breathe out as you stretch forward and breathe in as you release the stretch.

59

Leg Stretch

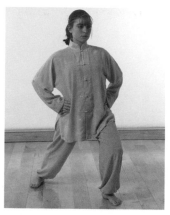

Stand with your legs apart, hands on hips. Step forward with your right leg, keeping your left leg straight. Do not bend your knee beyond your front foot. Repeat with your left leg.

Raising the Knee and Turning to the Side

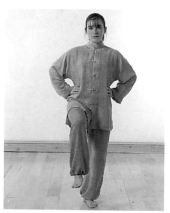

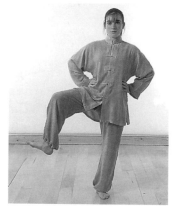

1 Stand with your legs apart, your hands on your hips. Slowly raise your right leg, so that your thigh is parallel to the floor.

2 Now turn your leg out from the hip, keeping your foot flexed (sole facing the floor) and lower your foot. Repeat the exercise with your left leg.

Tapping the Waist to clear the Belt Channel

In Chinese medicine, it is thought that tapping and rubbing parts of your body with your hands and fingers stimulates the healthy flow of Chi around the body.

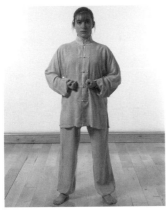

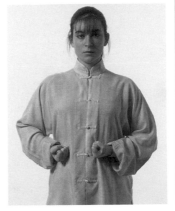

1 Hold your fists in front of your body.

2 Pull your right fist to the side.

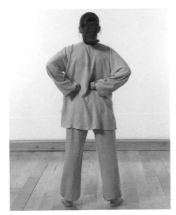

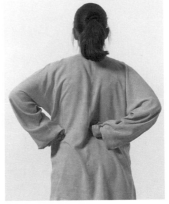

3 Place your right fist on your back and tap lightly six times.

4 Do the same with your left fist. Repeat the sequence starting with your left fist.

61

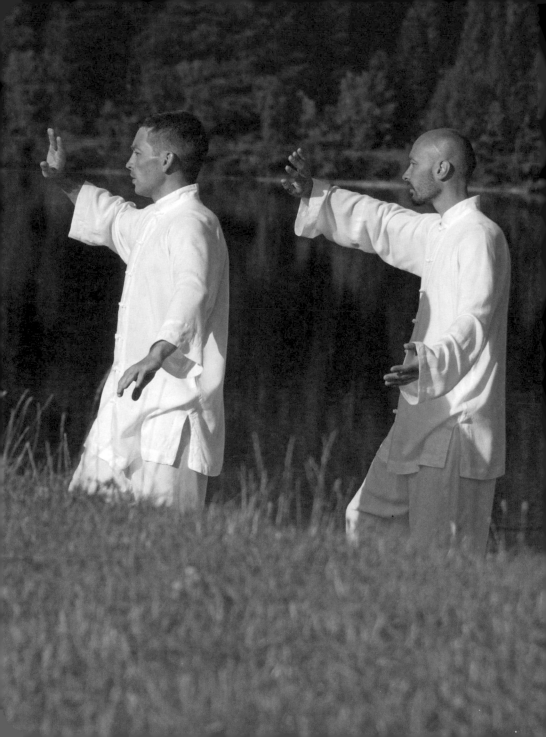

Chi Kung

This eighteen-step sequence of movements
introduces the idea of focusing the mind
on the flow of Chi as it enters, and
moves around, the body.

Chi Kung – Healing Mind

'The mind mobilises the Chi; the Chi mobilises the body.' Even in the first stages of practice, you will sense the movements of your Chi during the Chi Kung exercises. Learn to recognise this feeling so that you can direct and store your energy.

Reservoirs of Chi are situated throughout the body, but one of the most important is 5 cm (2 in) below your navel in an area called the Tan Tien in Chinese. When you practise Chi Kung, the following visualisation will help focus your mind:

Imagine that your hips and pelvis are a large sphere on which your upper body rests and from which your legs extend. As you breathe in, the air and Chi that you draw in with it fills the sphere; as you breathe out, the air, now carrying toxins and waste products, is expelled, leaving only a few drops of Chi at the very bottom of the sphere. Over time, as you practise this visualisation, the sphere will get fuller and heavier, anchoring you to the ground, but without ever weighing you down.

Chi Kung is the Chinese equivalent to Yoga. The literal translation of Chi Kung is 'Energy work'. Like Tai Chi, the movements of Chi Kung are soft, slow, circular and relaxed. Indeed, many authorities consider Tai Chi to be a style of Chi Kung. In any case, the practice of Chi Kung and Tai Chi go hand in hand.

The following eighteen Chi Kung exercises can be practised individually or as a continuous sequence (like the Tai Chi Form, see pages 98–157). If you are performing the exercises singly, you may repeat them from three to six times each. If you wish to perform them as a sequence, follow the instructions given in the introduction to each exercise in the 'sequence transition' section.

Unless otherwise stated in the instructions, while performing the Chi Kung exercises, your fingers should be extended in a natural curve and not stretched or held in a fist. Keep the thumb in line with your fingers.

Starting Position

This exercise will improve your mental functions and balance the flow of Chi in your body.

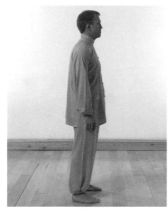

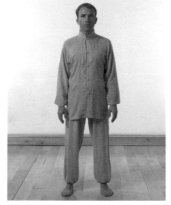

1 Stand with your feet shoulder-width apart, toes forward, knees soft. Hold your head and upper back straight, with your shoulders relaxed, and arms hanging loosely at your sides.

2 Breathe in and visualise the flow of air and Chi into your lungs and then down into your Tan Tien. Allow all the tension to leave your body as you breathe out.

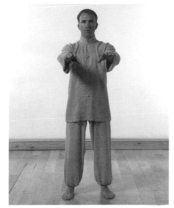

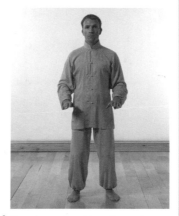

3 Take a long, slow breath in, and raise your arms to shoulder height. Keep the elbows and wrists soft but do not allow them to flop or hang.

4 Breathe out and bend your knees. If repeating the exercise, lower the arms and straighten your knees.

Opening the Chest

This exercise stimulates your heart-lung function and is beneficial to those suffering from breathing problems, such as asthma.

Sequence Transition

From Step 3 on page 65, instead of lowering the arms, keep them at shoulder height, breathe out, and straighten the knees. Turn your arms so that the palms of your hands face one another. Bend the elbows and bring the arms toward your chest. Go straight to Step 2 on this page.

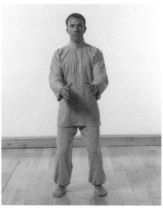

1 Stand in shoulder-width stance, with your knees slightly bent. Raise your arms to chest height, your palms facing one another.

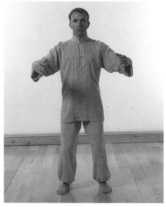

2 Breathe in and separate your arms, opening the chest and straightening your legs.

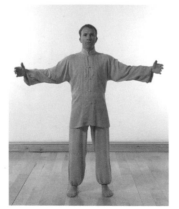

3 Expand your chest as much as possible as you reach full extension with your arms.

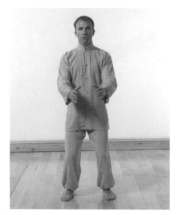

4 Breathe out and bend the knees as you bring the arms back to the centre of the body and then lower them to the sides.

Rainbow Dance

This exercise will correct poor posture in your upper back and shoulders by gently stretching your joints and muscles.

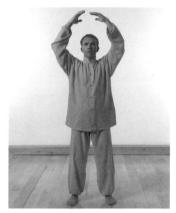

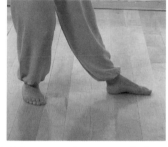

1 From the starting position stance, raise both hands in the front of your chest. Breathe in, straighten the legs and bring both hands over your head, palms facing each other.

2 Shift your weight to your right foot. Raise your left heel off the floor so that only the ball and toes are in contact with the floor. Breathe out and turn your body to the right.

Sequence Transition

In Step 4 on page 66, instead of dropping your arms all the way down, turn your palms to face one another. Breathe in and raise your arms over your head. Go straight to Step 2 on this page.

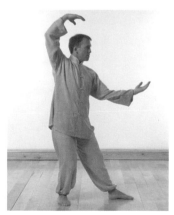

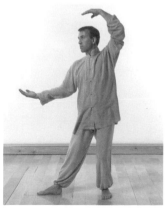

3 Breathe in as you bring your left hand down to shoulder height, palm facing up. Your right hand moves up so that your palm is directly over the top of your head.

4 Breathe out, turn to the left and return to the centre and reverse the direction of the exercise. It helps to imagine that you are holding a ball between your hand and head.

67

Separating Clouds by Wheeling Arms

This exercise will prevent arthritis in your knee and shoulder joints. It is also beneficial to your respiratory system.

Sequence Transition
On completing Step 4 on page 67, draw your feet back to the starting position with your weight on both feet, before moving on to Step 1 on this page.

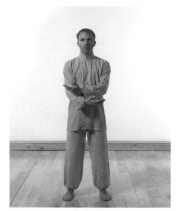

1 In the starting position stance, cross your arms in front of your body, with your left hand over your right. Breathe out and bend your knees.

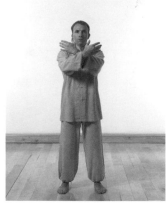

2 Breathe in as you raise your arms toward your head, straightening your knees.

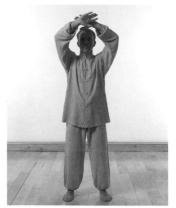

3 Open your arms as they rise above your head.

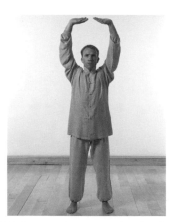

4 Make an arch over your head with your arms, and rotate your palms so that they face outward.

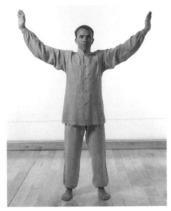

5 Breathe out and begin to lower your arms gently.

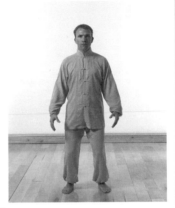

6 As you lower your arms, bend your knees slightly.

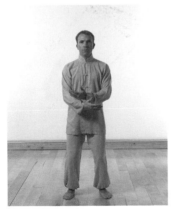

7 Finish with your arms crossed in front of you.

'When the spirit is raised, there is no fault of stagnancy and heaviness.'

Wu Yuxiang

69

Rolling Arms

This movement provides general benefits for the joints and muscles of your upper body and improves your breathing function.

Sequence Transition
From Step 7 on page 69, breathe in as you make the transition to Step 1 on this page.

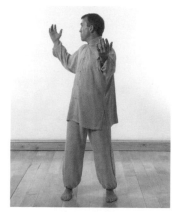

1 Stand with your left hand stretched out, palm up, at chest height. Raise your right hand, with your elbow bent, until it is level with your ear.

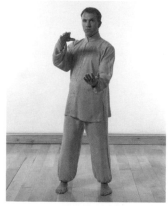

2 Breathe out as you move your right hand forward and down, and pull back your left hand, so that your palms cross in front of your chest.

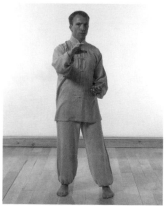

3 Breathe in as you turn your waist to the left, and shift your weight to your right foot, and stretch out your arms.

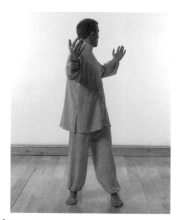

4 Breathe out as you draw your hands back so they cross in front of your chest. Turn your waist to the right. Shift your weight to your left foot. Breathe in as you stretch your arms.

Rowing the Boat in the Centre of the Lake

This exercise is beneficial to the joints of your shoulders, elbows and wrists, and improves your digestive function.

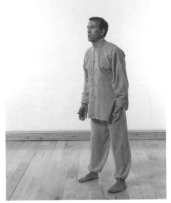

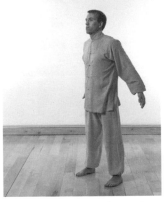

1 Stand relaxed in the starting position stance. Breathe in.

2 Bring your arms straight up from the side to the front and around over the top of your head.

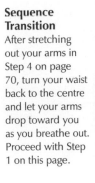

Sequence Transition
After stretching out your arms in Step 4 on page 70, turn your waist back to the centre and let your arms drop toward you as you breathe out. Proceed with Step 1 on this page.

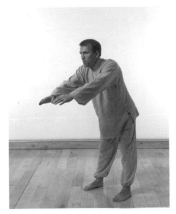

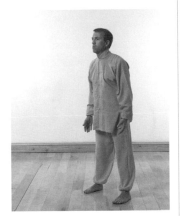

3 Breathe out and bend forward as your hands come around and down. Keep your arms straight and your palms facing down.

4 Straighten your body and return to the starting position stance.

71

Lifting the Ball in Front of the Shoulder

In addition to improving breathing, this exercise will work your shoulder joints and help with lower back and neck problems.

Sequence Transition

Remain in the finishing position of Step 4 on page 71, standing upright and with your arms and legs relaxed. Proceed with Step 1 on this page.

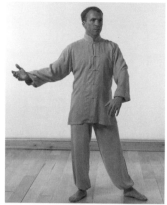

1 Standing in the starting position stance, raise your right hand, palm facing up, as if you are holding an imaginary ball.

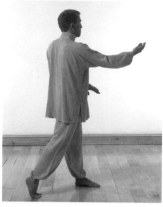

2 Turn your waist to the left and lift your right foot to your toes, turning it as you shift your weight onto your left foot. Breathe in as you draw your right arm up and across your body.

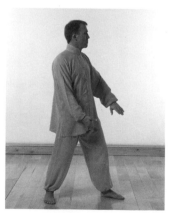

3 As you breathe out, turn your right palm face down and lower it. Turn and lower your right foot and return to the starting position. Repeat the whole movement with your left arm.

Pushing Palms While Turning the Waist

This movement is particularly beneficial to the spine, and is recommended for people who suffer from lower-back problems.

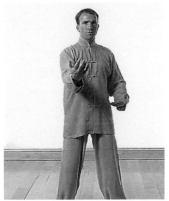

1 In starting position – hands at your waist, palms up – draw back your left hand, turn your waist to the left, and push forward with your right palm.

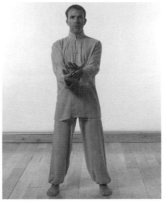

2 Breathe in. Draw the right hand back as you move your weight back to the centre. Your palms cross facing one other.

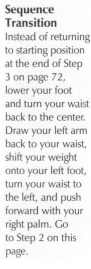

Sequence Transition

Instead of returning to starting position at the end of Step 3 on page 72, lower your foot and turn your waist back to the center. Draw your left arm back to your waist, shift your weight onto your left foot, turn your waist to the left, and push forward with your right palm. Go to Step 2 on this page.

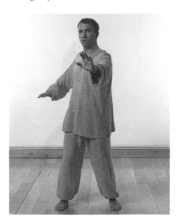

3 Shift your weight to the right foot and turn your waist to the right. Breathe out as your left palm pushes forward.

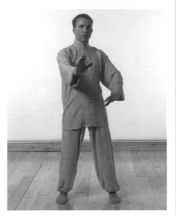

4 Shift your weight to the left foot and turn your waist to the left. Breathe out as your right palm pushes forward.

73

Cloud Hands in Horse Stance

This exercise will improve your mental and breathing functions. It is recommended for those with shoulder and lower-back problems.

Sequence Transition

Following Step 4 on page 73, allow your arms to drop slowly to your sides as you shift your weight to the centre so that you are supported equally by both feet. Bend your knees and raise both hands to your waist. This position is called the 'horse stance'. In the horse stance, your weight is evenly distributed between both feet, shoulder-width apart, and your knees bent, as if sitting astride a horse.

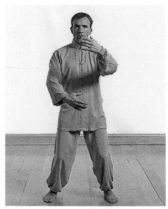

1 In horse stance, raise your left hand, palm facing you, level with your head, and bring your left hand, palm facing you, to waist height.

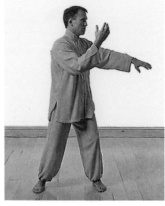

2 Turn your waist to the left. Lower your left hand, palm out then down. Raise your right hand, palm facing you. Allow your elbow to bend.

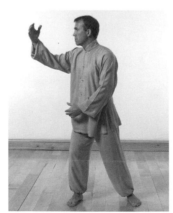

3 Turn your waist to the right, bringing your right hand in front of your face, and dropping your left hand across your body. Now perfor the mirror image of step 2.

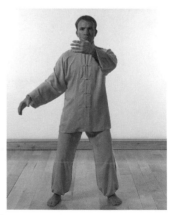

4 In effect, you are drawing two linked circles in front of you with your hands as you shift your weight from one foot to the other.

Looking at the Moon by Turning the Body

The turning motion of this exercise is beneficial to the entire spinal area, from the lower-back to the neck.

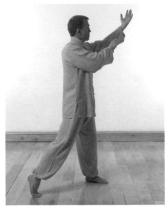

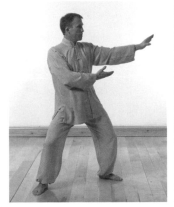

Sequence Transition
From Step 4 on page 74, allow your weight to settle in the centre, lower your arms to your sides and relax the shoulders, elbows and wrists. Proceed with Step 1 on this page.

1 Stand with arms at your sides. Turn to the left, shifting your weight to your left foot. Inhale as you swing both arms up.

2 Allow your right elbow to bend. Breathe out as you bend your knees, turn your waist to the centre and lower your arms.

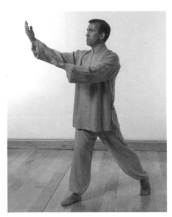

3 Repeat the movement turning to the right, breathing in as your body rises and out as it lowers.

75

Punching in Horse Stance

This exercise, borrowed from 'hard' kung fu styles, such as karate, is used in Tai Chi to develop internal as well as external strength.

Sequence Transition

On completion of Step 3 on page 75, lower the arms and turn the waist to the centre. Draw your arms to waist height, elbows bent, hands held in soft fists. Bend your knees and adopt the horse stance. Proceed with Step 1 on this page.

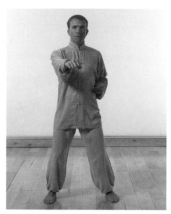 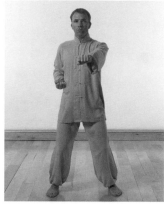

1 Stand in the horse stance, with your fists at waist height. Punch with your right arm, twisting the fist so that it finishes palm down.

2 Breathe out as you pull back your right hand and prepare to punch with your left hand. Breathe in as your fist completes the punch.

'When the left side is heavy, it empties and the right side is already countering. The Chi is like a wheel, and the whole body must coordinate.'

LI YUYU

Scooping the Sea While Looking at the Sky

The forward and backward bending movements of this exercise are beneficial to the spine, while massaging the internal organs.

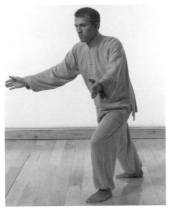

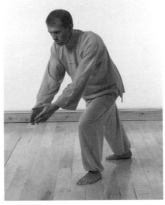

1 From the starting position stance, take a bow step to the left (see right for description) and stretch your arms in front of you.

2 Lean forward, bringing both hands together in front of your left knee. Bend your left knee but do not allow it to go over the toes of your left foot.

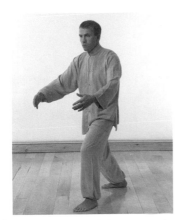

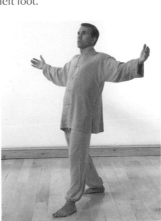

3 As you begin to shift your weight from your left to your right foot, draw your arms back and open them out to the sides.

4 Breathe in and look up as you open your arms wide. Return to the starting position and repeat the steps, this time taking a bow step to the right.

Sequence Transition

From Step 2 on page 76, open your hands and stretch both arms in front of you. Go to Step 2 on this page.

Left bow step: step out to the left with your left foot, toes pointing out, and shift your weight onto it so that it bends. Your right knee remains straight. See also page 42 'Bow Stance'.

Pushing Wave

A good exercise for the joints of the entire body, which will also improve your coordination. An extremely relaxing movement.

Sequence Transition
Remain in the right bow stance of Step 4 on page 77, shift your weight back so you are supported by both feet, and draw your arms to the side of your body, palms facing out. Go to Step 2 on this page.

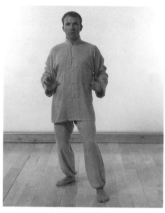

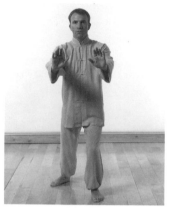

1 Step into the bow stance (see page 77) with your left foot. Lift your hands to your sides, both palms facing out.

2 Put your weight onto your left foot and push forward with your hands. Breathe out and stretch the back leg and lift your right heel off the floor.

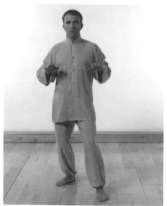

3 Slowly move your weight to your right leg. Breathe in and pull your arms back. Repeat the movement with a right bow stance.

Flying Pigeon

If you suffer from breathing problems, this movement may be of benefit to you because it regulates the respiratory, digestive and circulatory functions.

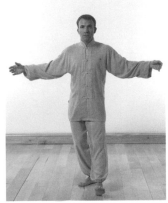

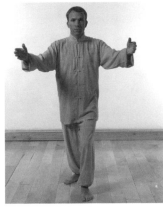

Sequence Transition
On completing Step 3 on page 78, shift your weight to your right foot, move your left foot to the right, toes pointing forward. Lift your arms to your side. Go to Step 2 on this page.

1 Step forward with your left foot. Lift up both arms to the sides. Breathe in and put your weight on your right foot. Lift up the toes of the left foot.

2 Breathe out and transfer your weight to your left foot, raising the heel of your right foot as you bring your hands together in front of your chest.

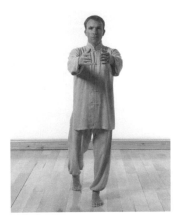

3 Pull back and repeat the exercise, stepping forward with your right foot.

Flying Wild Goose

This exercise is recommended to relax after a stressful day; it will also improve your respiratory function.

Sequence Transition

From Step 3 on page 79, lower your arms to your sides and step forward so that you are standing in horse stance. Draw your arms slightly away from your body, but keep them relaxed, with the joints soft and rounded. Go to Step 2 on this page.

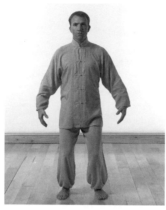

1 Stand in horse stance (see page 74), with your arms slightly apart from your sides, palms facing in.

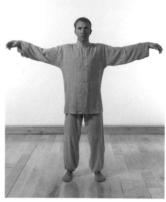

2 Breathe in as you straighten your knees and raise both arms out to the side.

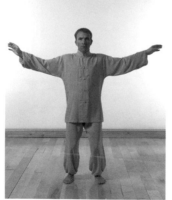

3 Stretch your hands in line with your arms, and begin to sink down.

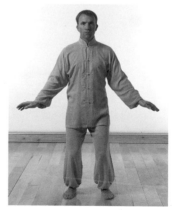

4 Breathe out as your hands drop and your knees bend.

Rotating Wheel in a Circle

This exercise is beneficial to the spine and will help people with lower-back problems.

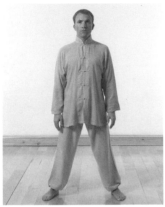

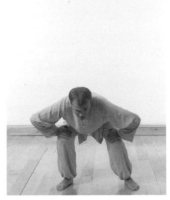

Sequence Transition
From Step 4 on page 80, continue to bend your knees until you are in a crouching position. Support the weight of your upper body with your hands on your thighs, fingers pointing inward. Go to Step 3 on page 82.

1 Stand with your feet slightly wider than shoulder width, with your arms by your sides.

2 Breathe out and bend forward, supporting your weight with your hands resting on your thighs. Your fingers should point inward.

'*Silently build up knowledge and turn it over in the mind.*'

WANG ZONYUE

Rotating Wheel in a Circle continued

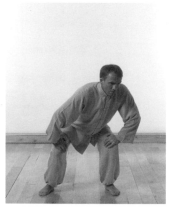

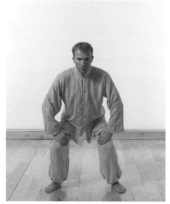

3 Rotate your body from your waist to the left until you have completed one full circle.

4 Breathe in as you rise to complete the circle. Keep your shoulders and back relaxed during the movement.

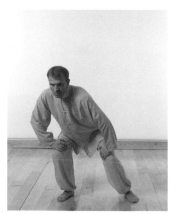

5 Return to the centre and repeat the circling motion to the right.

Marching While Bouncing Ball

This exercise strengthens many of the internal organs and can be used in cases of indigestion and other digestive problems.

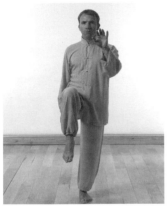

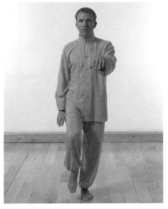

Sequence Transition
On completing Step 5 on page 82, straighten your knees, raise your right foot by bending your knee, and lift your left hand to shoulder height, palm facing forward. Go to Step 2 on this page.

1 Raise your right foot, toes relaxed, and lift your left hand to shoulder height, palm forward.

2 Breathe out and imagine you are bouncing a ball, as you lower your leg and hand.

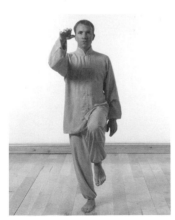

3 Breathe in as you raise your left leg and right arm, bouncing the ball with your left hand.

Shau Gong (Balancing Chi)

The concluding exercise in the sequence will balance the flow of Chi in your body. It is recommended for ailments of the digestive system.

Sequence Transition
From Step 3 on page 83, lower your arm and leg. Breathe in and turn your arms to the side, palms facing up. Go to Step 2 on this page.

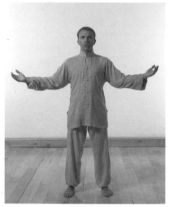

1 Stand in the starting position stance. Breathe in and raise your arms to the side, palms facing upward.

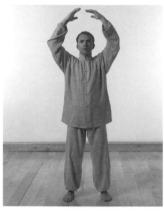

2 When your arms are above your head, your palms face downward, in front of your head.

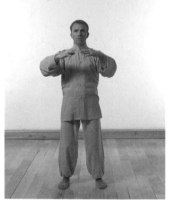

3 Breathe out and lower your arms along the front of your body.

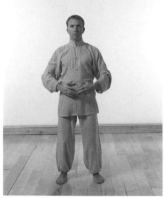

4 Bring your arms down to your stomach. Keep the shoulders, elbows and wrists soft and rounded.

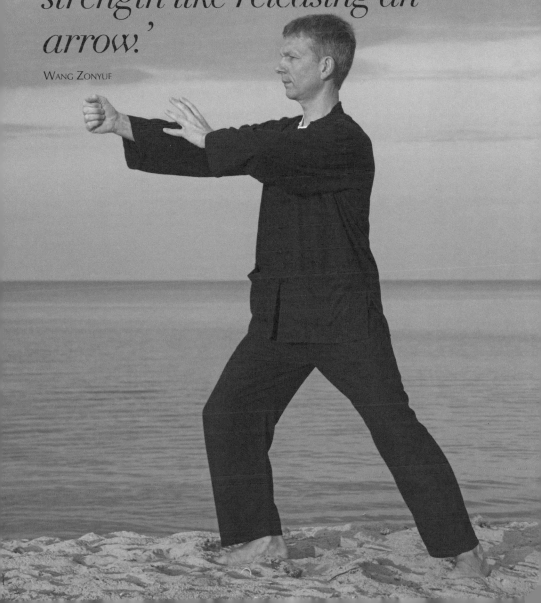

'*Store up the strength like drawing a bow. Release the strength like releasing an arrow.*'

WANG ZONYUF

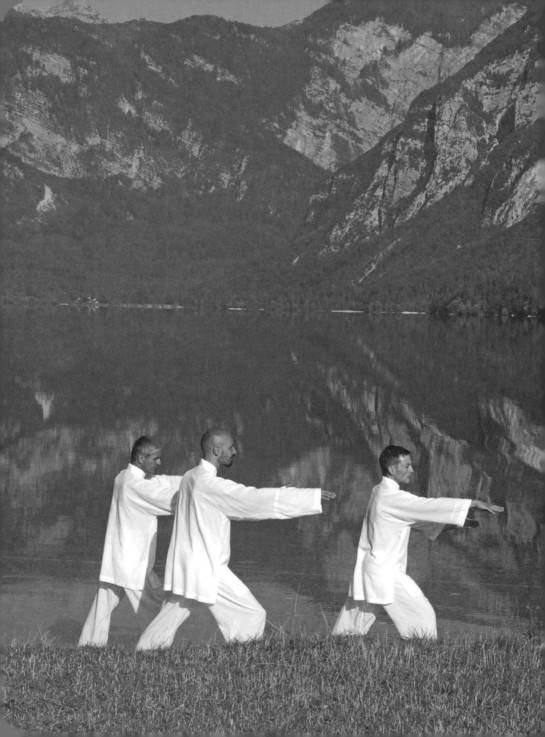

Six-method Chi Kung

These movements provide an excellent way of practising when you are short of time. Instead of trying to select a handful of movements from the full Chi Kung program, work through the steps that follow.

Six-method Chi Kung

Do not be disheartened if there are days when work or family responsibilities prevent you from completing the full warm-up and Chi Kung sequence. That is only natural. But rather than doing no practice at all, perform as many of the Chi Kung exercises as possible, without rushing them, in the time available to you. Alternatively, you may use the Six-method Chi Kung, which provides a short, comprehensive sequence of exercises to increase and regulate your Chi.

Gathering the Chi

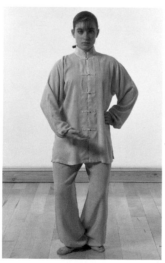 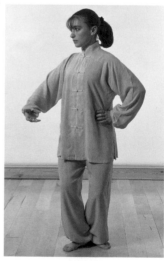

1 Stand with your right foot at right angles to your left foot, with both knees slightly bent. Rest your left hand on your hip and hold your right hand below your navel, palm facing up.

2 Turn to the right from the waist (and not the shoulders) and raise your hand upward and outward in a broad arc.

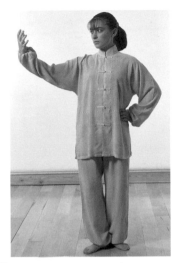

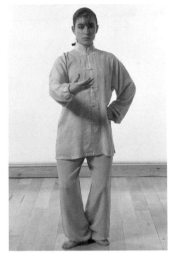

3 Breathe in and straighten your knees, until your right hand reaches head height, palm facing you.

4 Breathe out, turn your waist to the centre, lower your right hand down the centre of your body, and bend your knees.

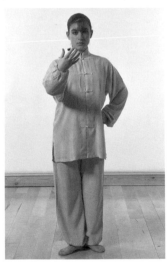

5 As you breathe in, imagine drawing the Chi into your hand. When you breathe out, imagine drawing the Chi down into the lower abdomen.

Crane Sips the Water

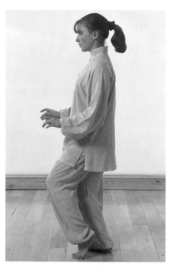 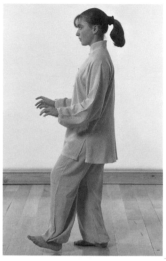

1 Stand with your weight on your right leg and bend your knees. Hold both hands out in front of you, both palms down.

2 Breathe out and slide your left foot, heel first, along the floor.

'Let the Chi move without breaks so that there is no part it cannot reach.'

WU YUXIANG

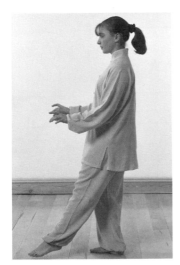

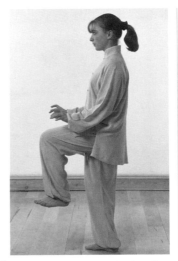

3 Breathe in, raise your left foot off the floor and lift your arms slightly.

4 Lift your foot higher by bending your left knee until your thigh is at a right angle to your body.

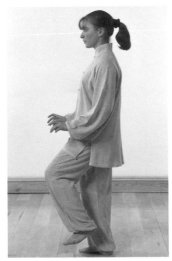

5 Return to the starting position and repeat the exercise with your weight resting on your left leg.

White Crane Spreads its Wings

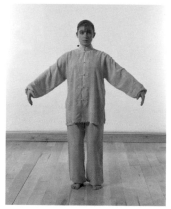 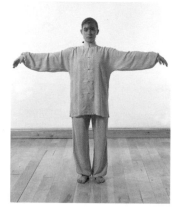

1 Stand with your feet slightly apart. Raise your arms to the sides, fingers, soft, hanging down.

2 Breathe in and continue raising your arms to shoulder height. Keep the fingers relaxed.

'A journey of a thousand leagues begins with but a single step.'

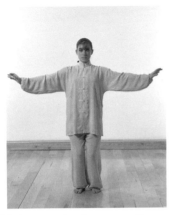 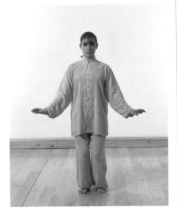

3 Raise your hands so your fingers point upward, breathe out, and bend the knees.

4 As you sink into the floor on bent knees, lower your arms, stretching your elbows and wrists.

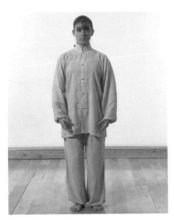

5 When your arms are at your sides, your palms should face inward. As you breathe in and out, imagine that the Chi is flowing to and from your hands through your palms.

Casting the Fishing Net

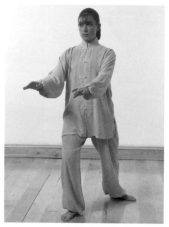

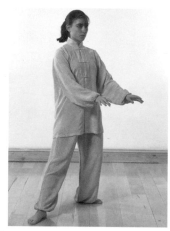

1 Stand with legs apart, knees slightly bent, the rear foot at right angles to the front foot. Hold your hands in front of you, palms facing down.

2 Shift your weight from your front to your rear foot. Then turn your waist in time with the forward and backward movement.

Dragon Chases the Moon

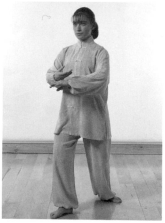

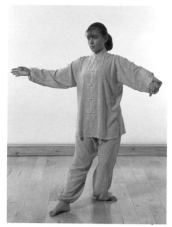

1 In the same stance as above, shift your weight forward and backward from your front to your rear foot.

2 With arms relaxed, circle both hands in a clockwise direction so that they cross at the centre of the body.

Dragon Swimming (Triple Rings)

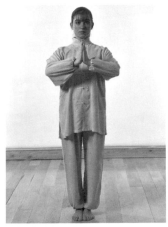

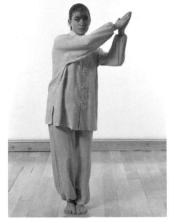

1 Stand with your feet and legs together. Press your palms together at chest height.

2 Raise your arms to the left, while twisting your legs and body to follow your hands.

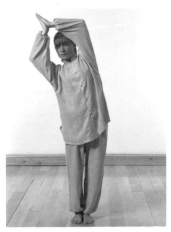

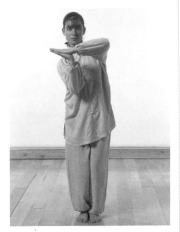

3 Make a circle above your head with your hands, leading your body to the right.

4 After circling your head, bend your knees and make a second circle to the left at chest height.

95

The Tai Chi Healing Bible

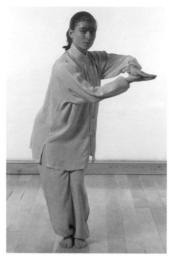

5 Twist the arms around so that the right arm remains lower than the left arm.

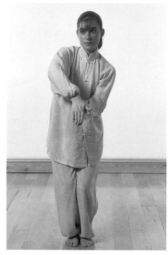

6 Bend your knees as you start the third and final circle at waist height. Twist to the right.

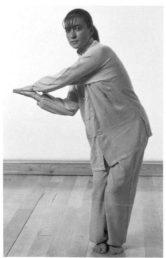

7 The final circle follows in the same direction, with your left arm uppermost.

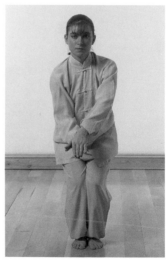

8 Double back to the centre of your body and complete the final circle.

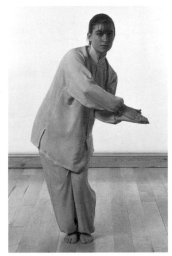

9 Move slowly and breathe evenly as you lower your body to the lowest point.

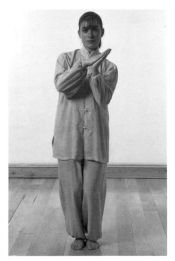

10 Repeat the three circles from your waist up in the opposite direction.

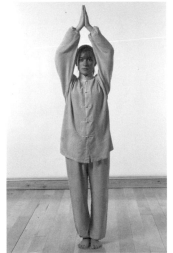

11 Finish with your legs straight and your hands clasped together over your head.

'If the body is clumsy then in advancing or retreating it cannot be free.'

Lɪ Yᴜʏᴜ

97

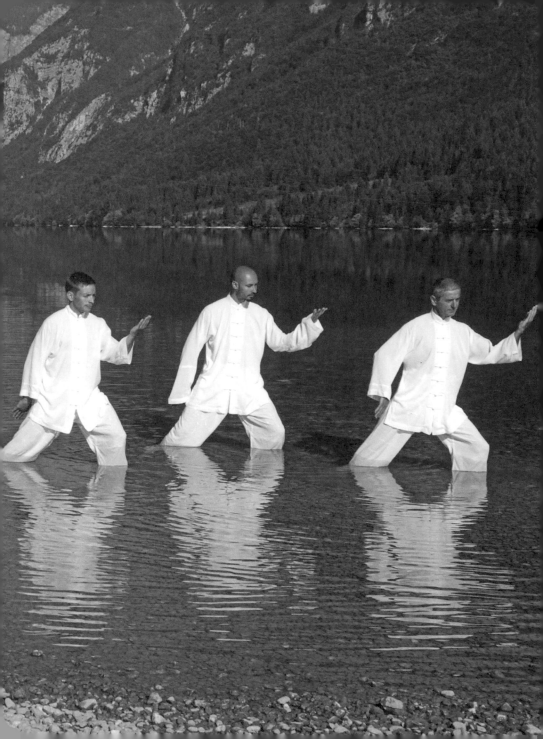

The Form

Having spent time practising the Chi Kung exercises in the previous chapters, you can now move on to the twenty-four-step Form. As you practise the movements, allow yourself to unite mind, body and spirit

Twenty-four-step Simplified Tai Chi Chuan

On the surface The Form appears to be no more than a sequence of punches, kicks and parries, which are common to many of the martial arts; but at a deeper level, the correct practice of The Form requires an understanding of breathing techniques, of the circulation of Chi, and of the focused single-pointed mind of meditation.

Many students are discouraged in the early stages of practice, because there seem to be so many elements to remember for each step. But you will quickly discover that many of the twenty-four steps are composed of shared movements of the feet, hands and waist. Approach your study of the form in stages. Learn and practise the first three steps only, and the the transitions that link them. When you have learned the first three steps, add another three, and work through all six. Carry on in this manner until you have covered the full twenty-four. Then you may concentrate on the other aspects of The Form, such as breathing and the circulation of Chi.

To help you work out which way you should be facing, imagine that you are standing in the centre of a clock face, looking toward 12 o'clock at the beginning of the form, with 3 o'clock on your right, and 9 o'clock on your left. The figure in each of the photographs shows the direction in which you should be looking as you complete the movement.

Step 1: Commencing Form

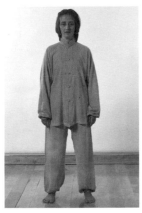

1 Facing 12 o'clock, stand with feet shoulder-width apart, toes forward, knees relaxed, and arms by your sides.

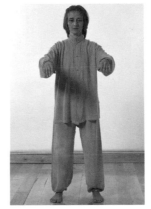

2 Breathe in and raise your arms, palms down, to shoulder height. Imagine the flow of Chi into your lungs.

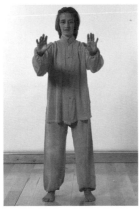

3 Keep shoulders and elbows soft and head straight as you breathe out. Press your palms down and bend your knees.

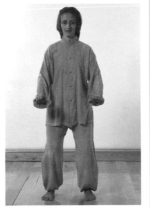

4 Lower your hands to hip height. Keep your knees bent with your weight distributed equally on both feet.

Step 2: Part Wild Horse Mane on Both Sides

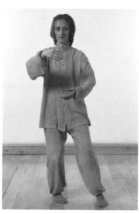

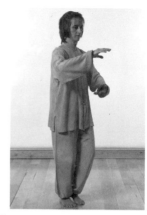

5 Turn to the right (to 1 o'clock) and shift your weight onto your right foot. Raise your right hand, palm down, to shoulder height.

6 Move your left hand, palm up, under your right hand, as if you were holding a ball in front of you. This is known as the 'hold-ball' gesture. Look at your right hand.

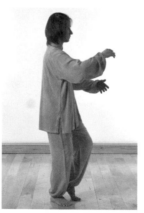

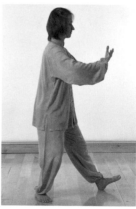

7 Lift your left foot and bring it next to your right foot, with your left heel off the floor.

8 Turn to the left and step into a left bow stance (see page 77) to face 8 o'clock. Put your left heel down first. Begin to push your left hand up and your right hand down.

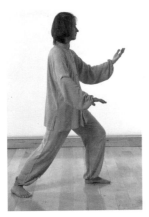

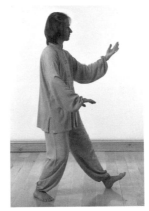

9 Shift your weight onto your left foot. Raise your left hand to eye level, palm facing up, and lower your right hand to your hip, palm facing down. You are facing 9 o'clock.

10 Move your weight back onto your right foot. Raise the toes of your left foot and turn them out (left) before putting your foot flat on the floor.

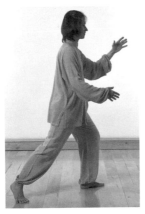

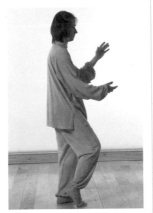

11 Shift your weight onto your left foot, and draw your hands into a hold-ball gesture in front of your left side with your left arm uppermost.

12 Complete the hold-ball gesture. Draw your right foot next to your left foot, with only your right toes on the floor. Look at your left hand.

103

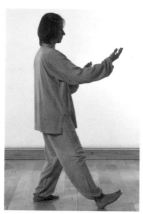

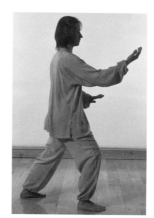

13 Move your weight onto your left foot. Turn right and step with your right foot to 10:30.

14 Complete the right bow stance. Turn your right toes out. Raise your right hand to eye level, and lower your left hand to your left hip. You are facing 9 o'clock.

Points to Remember

- The parting the mane action occurs three times in total.
- Hold your upper body upright, as if your head were suspended by a thread, and keep your chest sunk.
- Your arm movements should be large and rounded.
- When you turn your body, turn from your waist and not from your shoulders.
- When you step forward, put your foot down slowly in position, with the heel touching first.
- Your leading knee should not go beyond the toes of the same foot, and your rear foot should be at a 45–60° angle to your front foot.

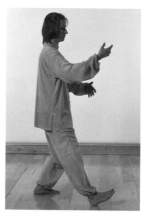

15 Shift your weight onto your left foot and sit back, raising the toes of your right foot off the floor and turning them out slightly.

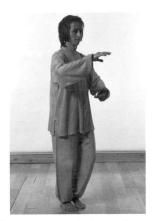

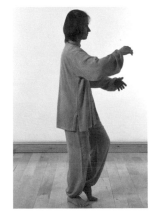

16 Lower your right foot and put your weight on it. Draw your left foot to your right foot, and make a hold-ball gesture in front of you, with your right arm on top.

17 The sequence then follows the same steps as the first part of the Horse Mane.

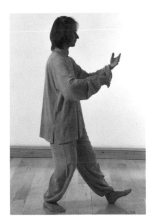

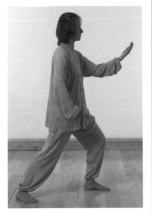

18 Shift your weight to your right foot, raising your left toes off the floor and sit back. Turn your body to the left and take a left bow step (to 8 o'clock).

19 Part the Horse's Mane, completing the left bow step to 8 o'clock, with your left hand raised at eye level and your right hand by your right hip. Look straight ahead.

105

Step 3: White Crane Spreads its Wings

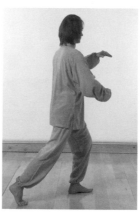 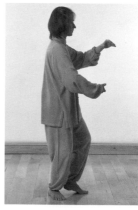

20 Shift all your weight onto your left foot. Turn to the left and make a hold-ball gesture in front of your left side, with the left hand on top. Look at your left hand.

21 Draw your right foot behind your left foot. Turn slightly to the right and look at your right hand. Sit back onto your right foot.

Points to Remember

- Do not stick your chest out.
- Your arms should be rounded when they move up or down.
- You should raise your right hand as you shift your weight back onto your right leg.
- Your left foot carries no weight, and your left knee is slightly bent.

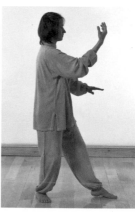

22 Move your left foot forward. Raise your right hand forward until level with your right temple, palm in. Lower your left hand, palm down. Look straight ahead.

Step 4: Brush Knee and Twist Step on Both Sides

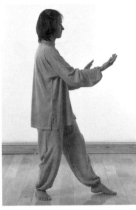

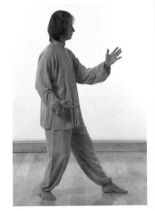

23 Remain in the empty stance and turn left to 8 o'clock. Your right hand moves down and your left hand up.

24 Turn to the right, your right hand moving down, palm up, past your face, while your left hand, palm down, circles up, stopping in front of your right side.

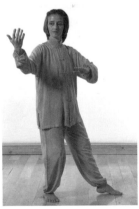

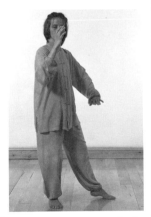

25 Turn to the left, prepare to take a left bow step to 8 o'clock. Draw your right hand left past your right ear.

26 After you turn your body, push your right hand forward at nose level, palm facing out, while your left hand drops and circles around your left knee.

107

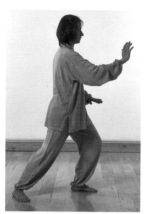

27 Complete the bow stance and stop your left hand beside your left hip, palm down. Look at the fingers of your extended right hand, palm out.

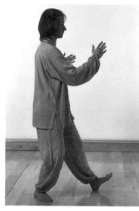

28 Shift your weight to your right foot, bending your right knee. Raise the toes of your left foot and turn them slightly out (left) before placing your foot flat on floor.

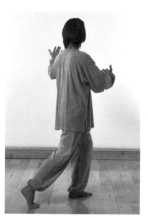

29 Bend your left leg. Turn your body to the left and shift your weight onto your left foot.

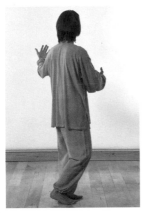

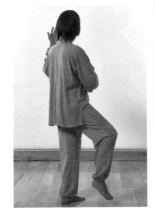

30 Bring your right foot next to your left, on its toes. Move your left hand, palm up, to shoulder height, and your right hand up, as you turn, then down to the left. Look at your left hand.

31 Take a right bow step to 10 o'clock. Draw your left hand past your left ear.

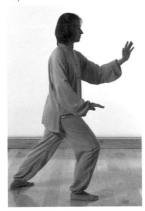

32 After you turn your body, push your left hand forward at nose level, palm facing out. Drop your right hand to stop beside your right hip. Look at your left hand.

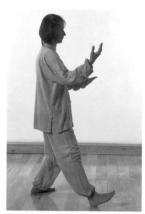

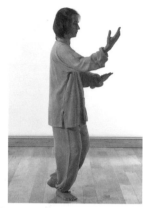

33 Shift your weight to your left foot, bending your left knee. Raise the toes of your right foot and turn them slightly out (right) before placing your foot flat on floor.

34 Bend your right leg. Turn to the right, shift your weight to your right foot. Move your left hand across your face, circle your right hand out and back to your ear.

Points to Remember

- You perform the brush knee sequence three times: to the left, right, and left again.
- Keep your upper body straight when you push your hands forward.
- Your waist and hips should be relaxed.
- Coordinate the movements of your hands with those of your waist and legs.
- The distance between your heels should be about 30 cm (12 in).

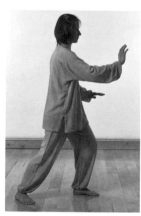

35 Make a left bow stance (to 8 o'clock) and circle your left hand down and stop by your left hip, palm facing down. Push the right hand until the arm is extended.

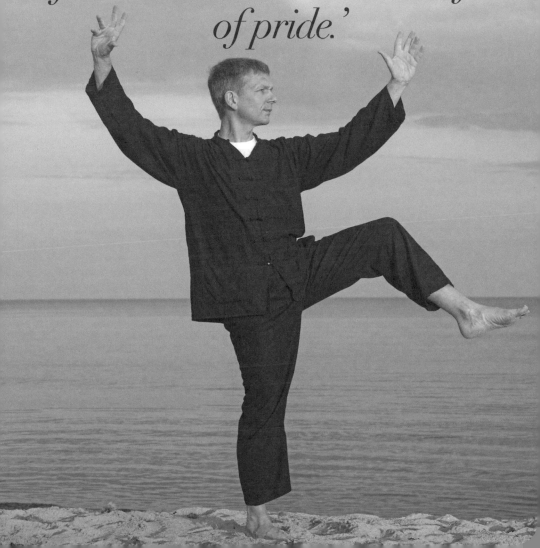

'Stand like a child who has learned to take its first steps, with your shoulders and neck free of tension and chest sunken, free of pride.'

Step 5: Hand Strums the Lute

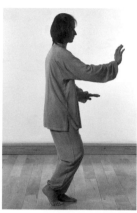

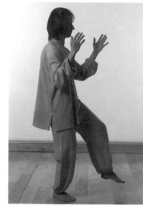

36 Take half a step with your right foot toward your left heel. Turn to the right slightly, and shift your weight onto your right foot.

37 As you turn, raise your left hand to nose level, palm facing right, elbow slightly bent. Circle your right hand opposite your left elbow, palm facing left. Raise your left foot.

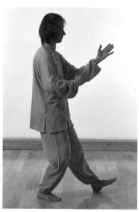

38 Complete the left empty stance by resting your left foot on its heel, but without shifting any weight onto it. Do not rise or fall as you move into the final position.

Step 6: Step Back to Drive Monkey Away

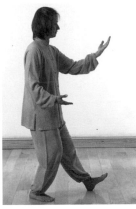

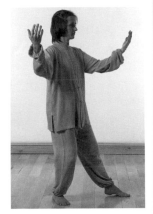

39 Turn slightly to the right. Lower your right hand, palm facing up, toward your hip in a circular motion.

40 Continue circling your right hand until it reaches shoulder level, with your palm facing up and your elbow slightly bent.

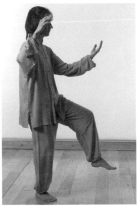

41 Bring your right hand to your right ear, and turn to the left. Push your right hand forward and your left hand down as you raise your left foot to step back.

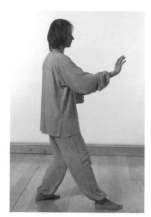

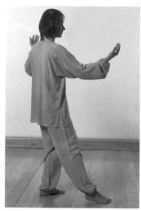

42 Place your left foot on the floor. Turn to the left and shift your weight onto your left foot to make a right empty stance, with your right foot pivoting on its toes until it points forward.

43 Bring your left hand level with your left ear and turn to the right. Push your left hand forward.

Points to Remember

- When pushing out or drawing back, move your hands in an arc – not in a straight line.
- While pushing out your hands, keep your waist and hips relaxed.
- Coordinate the turning of your waist with your hand movements.

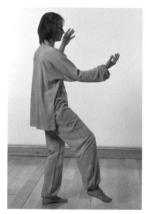

44 As your hands move, raise your right foot and step back as before, this time shifting your weight to the right foot. Look at your left hand (to 9 o'clock).

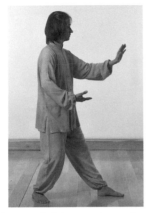

45 Turn slightly to the right. Lower your right hand toward your hip in a circular motion.

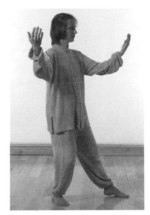

46 Continue circling your right hand until it reaches shoulder level with your palm facing up and your elbow slightly bent.

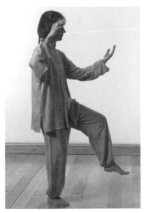

47 Bring your right hand to your right ear and turn to the left. Push your right hand forward and the left down by your waist as you step back with your left foot.

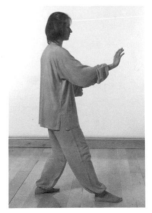

48 Place your foot slowly in position. Turn your body to the left and shift your weight onto your left foot to form an empty step. Look at your right hand (to 9 o'clock).

115

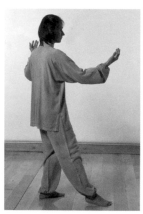

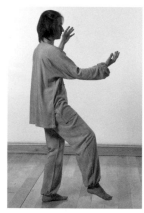

49 Bring your left hand level with your ear and turn to the right. Push your left hand forward.

50 As your hands move, raise your right foot and step back as before, this time shifting your weight to the right foot.

Points to Remember

- You step back four times: with your left foot, right foot, and left and right again.
- When stepping back, place your toes down first and then set the entire foot on the floor.
- Turn your front foot simultaneously with the body turn, pivoting on your toes, until the foot comes in line with your body.
- Move your left leg slightly toward the left – or right leg slightly toward the right, as the case may be – when taking a step backward, being careful not to let the feet land in a straight line.

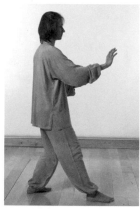

51 Bring your left hand level with your ear and turn to the right. Push your left hand forward.

Step 7: Grasp the Bird's Tail – Left Style

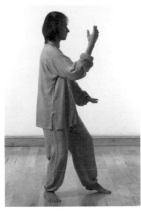

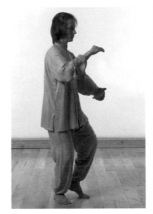

52 Turn to the right. Move your right hand up and to the side, to shoulder height, palm facing up, while your left hand is palm down. Look at your left hand.

53 Make a hold-ball in front of your right side, with your right hand on top. Shift your weight onto your right foot, draw your left foot, on its toes, next to your right foot.

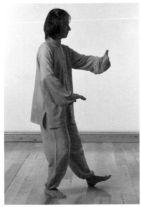

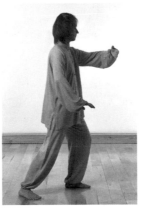

54 Turn your body slightly to the left, raise your left foot and step forward.

55 Turn a little more to the left, and complete the left bow stance. Push out your left forearm, palm in. Drop your right hand by your right hip, palm down.

117

The Tai Chi Healing Bible

Points to Remember

• Keep the upper body erect when pressing the hands forward; coordinate the movement of your hands with the relaxing of your waist and the bending of your leg.

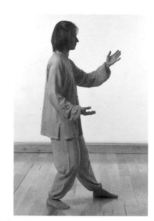

56 Shift your weight to your right foot. Turn to the left, stretching your left hand forward, palm down. Bring your right hand up, palm turning upward, until below your left forearm.

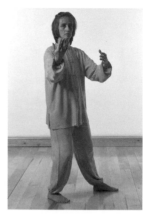

57 Turn to the right, drawing your hands in an arc in front of you. Finish with your right hand extended at shoulder height, palm up, and the left across your chest, palm in.

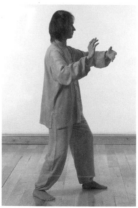

58 Shift your weight onto the right foot. Look at your right hand. Turn slightly to the left. Bend your right arm and place your right hand inside your left wrist.

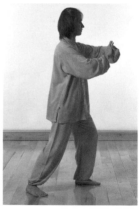

59 Turn further to the left. Press both hands forward, right palm facing out and left palm facing in. Shift your weight onto your left foot to make a left bow stance.

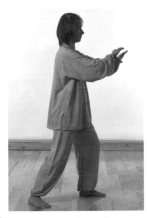

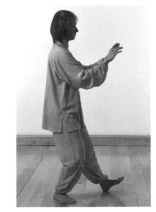

60 Turn both palms down as your right hand passes over your left wrist and moves forward and to the right, ending level with your left hand.

61 Open your hands shoulder-width apart, and shift your weight onto your right foot, left toes lifted. Pull your hands in front of you, palms out and slightly down.

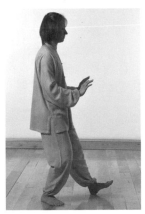

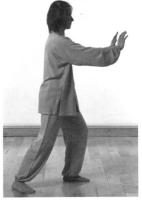

62 Lower both your hands to your waist. Do not lower them in a straight line, but in an S-shaped movement.

63 Shift your weight onto your left foot, making a left bow stance. Push your hands forward and up, palms out, until your wrists are at shoulder height.

119

Step 8: Grasp the Bird's Tail – Right Style

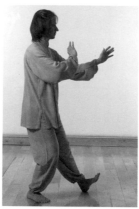

64 Sit back, shifting your weight onto your right foot, and lift your left toes.

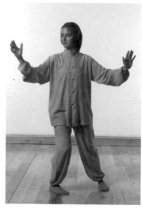

65 Turn to the right and pivot the toes of your left foot in. Move your right arm to the right. Turn the left palm out.

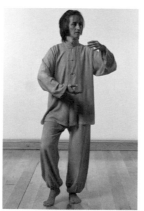

66 Move your right hand past up to your left ribs, palm up, forming a hold-ball gesture with your left hand on top. Shift your weight back onto your left foot.

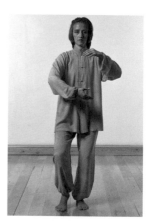

67 Place your right foot beside your left foot, with its heel raised. Look at your left hand.

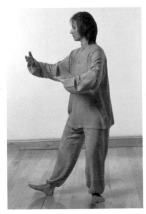

68 Turn to the right (to 3 o'clock). Take a step to the right (4 o'clock) with your right foot, placing your foot down heel first.

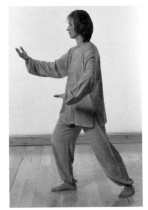

69 Shift your weight onto your right leg. Push out your right forearm, palm in. Drop your left hand by your left hip, palm down, fingers forward.

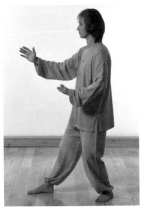

70 Turn to the right, stretching your right hand, palm down, Raise your left hand, palm turning up, until it is below your right forearm.

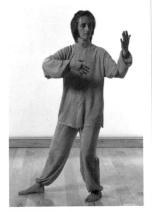

71 Turn to the left. Draw your hands in an arc – left hand to shoulder height, palm up, right forearm across your chest, palm in. Shift your weight onto your left foot.

121

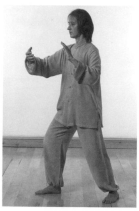

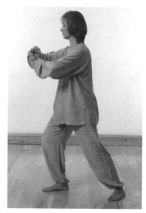

72 Turn slightly to the right. Bend your left arm and place your left hand inside your right wrist.

73 Turn a little further to the right. Press both hands forward, with left palm facing out and right palm facing in. Shift your weight onto your right foot to take a right bow stance.

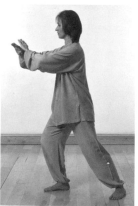

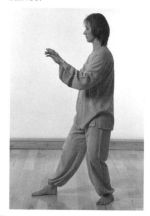

74 Turn both your palms down as your left hand passes over your right wrist and moves forward and to the left, ending level with your right hand.

75 Open your hands shoulder-width apart, palms turning out and down. Sit back onto your left foot, with your right toes raised off the floor.

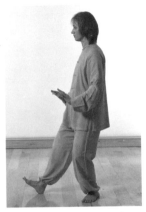

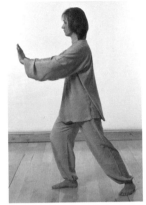

76 Draw your palms down from chest to waist height.

77 Shift your weight onto your right foot, making a right bow stance. Push your hands forward and up, palms facing forward until your wrists are at shoulder height. You are facing 3 o'clock in the final position.

'Move through the form at a constant pace, as if you were swimming on dry land, your limbs and head buoyed up by the universal Chi.'

123

Step 9: Single Whip

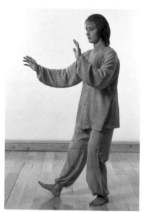 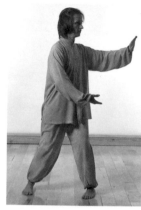

78 Sit back and shift your weight onto your left foot and turn in the toes of your right foot.

79 Turn your body to the left. Move your hands left, with your left hand on top, until your left arm is stretched at shoulder height, palm facing out, and your right hand is in front of your left ribs, palm tilted in. Look at your left hand (to 10 o'clock).

Points to Remember

- Keep your upper body straight and your waist relaxed.
- Bend your right elbow slightly down and have your left elbow directly above your left knee.
- Lower your shoulders.
- Turn out your left palm in time as you press your left hand forward.

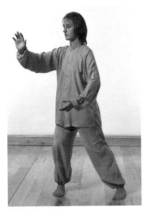

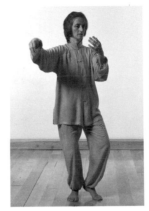

80 Turn to the right, weight on your right foot. Draw your left foot on its toes next to your right foot. Arc your right hand up until your arm is at shoulder height.

81 With the right palm turned out, bunch your fingertips and turn them down from the wrist to form a 'hooked hand'.

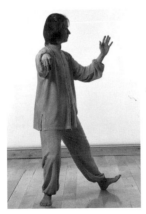

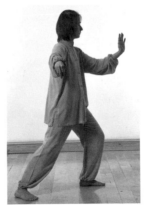

82 Turn your body to the left, facing 9 o'clock, and take a step forward with your left foot (to 8 o'clock), heel first.

83 Your left arm moves left at eye level, the palm turning out as it sweeps across, Step into a left bow stance. Look at your left hand (to 9 o'clock).

Step 10: Wave Hands Like Clouds – Left Style

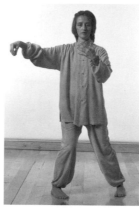

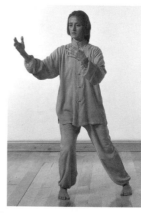

84 Shift your weight onto your right foot. Turn to the right, turning the toes of your left foot in. Make an arc with the left hand, finishing in front of your right shoulder, palm tilted in.

85 At the same time, open your hooked right hand and turn the palm out. Look at your right hand (to 3 o'clock).

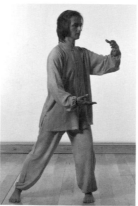

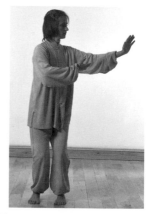

86 Turn to the left, shifting your weight onto your left foot. Make an arc past your face with your left hand, turning your left palm out. Look at your left hand.

87 Your right hand makes an arc past your abdomen and then up to your left shoulder, with the palm tilted in.

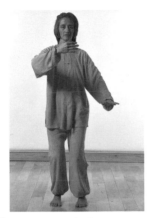

88 Bring your right foot next to your left foot so that your feet are in parallel stance, and about 10–20 cm (4–8 in) apart.

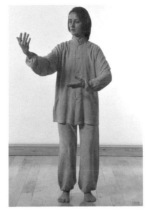

89 Turn to the right and shift your weight onto your right foot. Look at your right hand (to 3 o'clock).

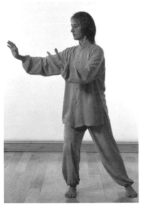

90 Your right hand continues to move right, past your face, palm out. Your left hand makes an arc up to shoulder level, palm in. Take a side step with your left foot.

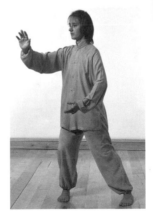

91 Shift your weight onto your right foot and turn your body to the right, while turning the toes of your left foot in. Make an arc with your left hand.

127

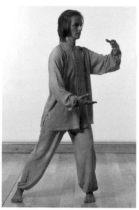

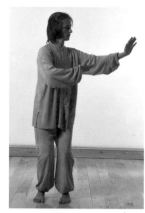

92 Turn to the left, shifting your weight onto your left foot. Make an arc past your face with your left hand, turning your left palm out.

93 Your right hand makes an arc past your abdomen and then up to your left shoulder, with the palm tilted in.

Points to Remember

- Your lower spine serves as the axis for the body turns.
- Keep your waist and hips relaxed and avoid a sudden rise or fall of body position.
- The movement of your arms should be relaxed and circular, and follow that of the waist.
- The pace must be slow and even.
- Keep your balance when moving your lower limbs.
- Follow the hand with your eyes when it moves past your face.

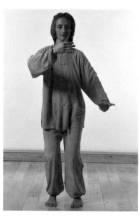

94 Bring your right foot to the side of your left foot, so that your feet are in parallel stance, about 10–20 cm (4–8 in) apart. Look at your right hand.

Step 11: Single Whip

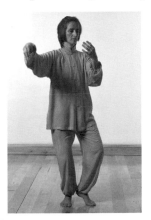

95 Turn to the right, move the right hand to the right side, hooked, just above shoulder height. Your left hand makes an arc up to your right shoulder, left palm in.

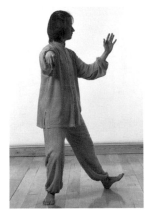

96 Turn your body to the left, facing 9 o'clock, and take a step forward with your left foot, heel touching the floor first (to 8 o'clock).

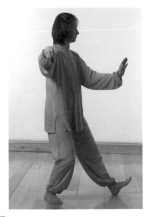

97 Slowly rotate your left palm and push your left arm ahead at eye level. Start shifting your weight onto your left foot.

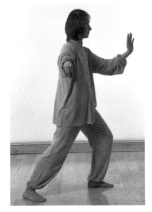

98 Complete the left bow stance. Look at your left hand (to 9 o'clock).

Points to Remember

- Keep your upper body straight and your waist relaxed.
- Bend your right elbow slightly down and have your left elbow directly above your left knee.
- Lower your shoulders.
- Turn out your left palm in time as you press your left hand forward.

129

Step 12: High Pat on Horse

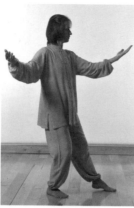 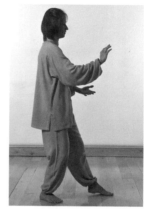

99 Take half a step forward with your right foot and shift your weight onto it. Open your right hook hand and turn both palms up, elbows slightly bent, while you turn slightly to the right, raising the left heel. Look ahead. Turn to the left (to 9 o'clock).

100 Draw your right hand past your right ear and push it forward, palm out, at eye level. Lower your left hand until it comes in front of your left hip, palm up. Bring your left foot forward, forming an empty stance. Look at your right hand.

Points to Remember

• Hold your upper body straight and relaxed. Keep your shoulders low and your right elbow slightly bent down. Do not let your body rise or fall when shifting your weight from your left to your right leg.

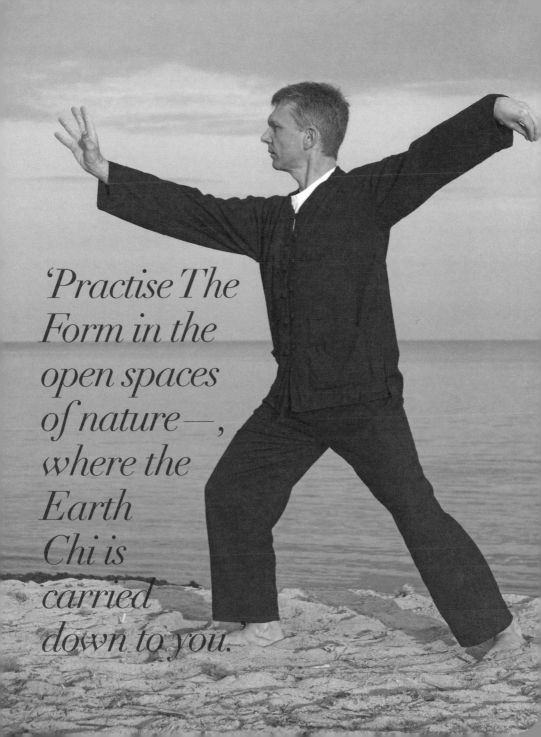

'Practise The Form in the open spaces of nature—, where the Earth Chi is carried down to you.'

Step 13: Kick with Right Heel

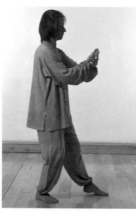 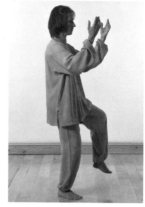

101 With your weight supported on your right foot, turn to the right (to 10 o'clock), and cross your left hand, palm in, over your right wrist, palm out.

102 Separate your hands, each making a downward circle with the palms tilted down. Raise your left foot to take a step forward (to 8 o'clock).

'Do not allow your body, mind and spirit to squabble, but fuse their efforts to achieve your goal.

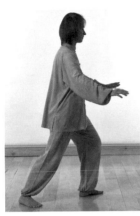

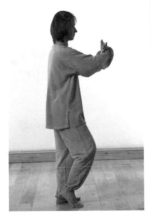

103 Place your left foot down to make a left bow stance, with your left toes slightly turned out. Look straight ahead. Continue to circle your hands out.

104 Bring your hands up until they cross in front of your chest, with your left hand over your right hand, palms in.

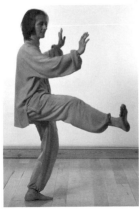

105 Open your arms to shoulder height, elbows bent and palms out. Raise your right leg, knee bent, and kick with your right foot (to 10 o'clock).

133

Step 14: Strike with Both Fists

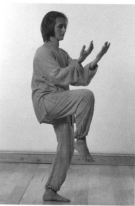

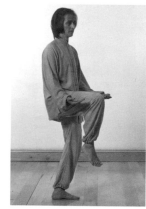

106 Pull back your right foot but keep your thigh parallel to the floor. Move your left hand up and forward, then down to the side of your right hand in front of your chest, turning both palms up.

107 Both arms, elbows soft, drop to either side of your right knee. Look straight ahead.

Points to Remember

- Hold your head and neck straight.
- Your fists are loosely clenched.
- Keep your shoulders relaxed, and allow your arms to move down naturally with your elbows slightly bent.

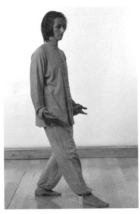

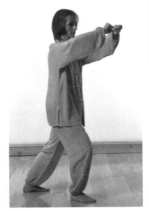

108 Put your right foot slightly forward and to the right. Shift your weight to your right foot to make a bow step. Drop both hands, fists loosely clenched.

109 Extend your fists up, as if punching someone on both ears, knuckles tilted up. The distance between your fists is about 10–20 cm (4–8 in).

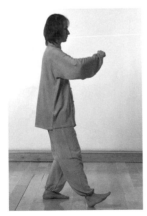

110 Bend your left leg and sit back. Turn your body to the left, toes of your right foot pointing in. Open your hands and move them out and down.

135

Step 15: Turn and Kick with Left Heel

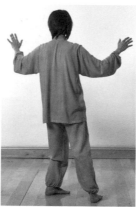 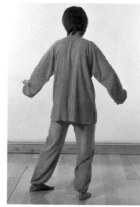

111 Continue to separate your hands, palms facing forward, in a circular movement. Straightening your arms at the elbow, look at your left hand.

112 Shift your weight onto your right foot. Bring your left foot next to it and rest its toes, and circle your hands downward and to the sides.

Points to Remember

- As in the right style, your wrists are level with your shoulders when you open your hands.
- Your right leg is slightly bent when your left foot kicks; the force of the kick comes from your heel, with the upturned toes pointing slightly in.
- Coordinate the separation of your hands with the kick.
- The left arm is parallel with the left leg.

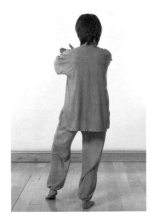

113 Continue circling in and forward, until your hands cross in front of your chest, with your right hand over your left hand, both palms facing in.

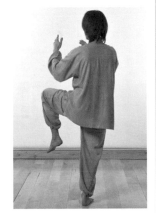

114 Raise your left foot off the floor and start to separate your hands to the side.

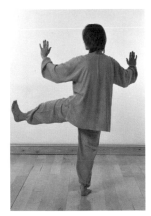

115 Open your arms to the side at shoulder level, elbows slightly bent and palms turning out. Kick with your left heel (to 4 o'clock).

137

Step 16: Squat Down and Stand on One Leg – Left Style

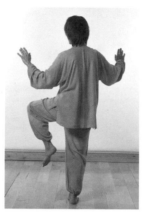

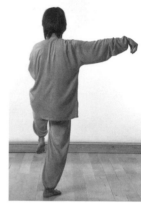

116 Pull back your left foot but keep it raised, with your thigh parallel to the floor.

117 Turn to the right. Make a right hooked hand. Your left palm turns up and makes an arc across your body until in front of your right shoulder, tilted in.

Points to Remember

- Raise your left foot slightly before crouching and stretching your left leg.
- Bend your standing leg slightly.
- Your toes should point naturally down as you raise your right foot.

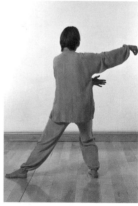

118 Turn left and bend your right knee, stretching your left leg to the side. Extend your left hand along the inner side of your left leg, palm forward.

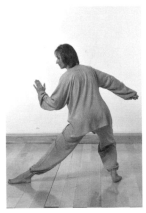

119 When your right leg is bent in a full crouch, turn the toes of your right foot out slightly and straighten your left leg with the toes turned in slightly.

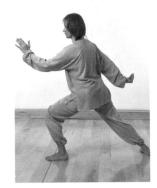

120 Turn the toes of your right foot in, straighten your right leg and bend your left. Extend your left arm forward and drop the right hand behind, fingers bent.

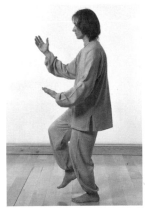

121 Raise your right foot until your right thigh is parallel to the floor.

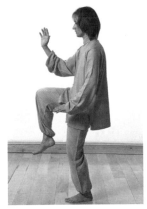

122 Swing your right hand up, until the elbow is just above your right knee, fingers up, palm left. Lower your left hand to your hip, palm down.

139

Step 17: Squat Down and Stand on One Leg – Right Style

Points to Remember

- Raise your right foot slightly before crouching and stretching your right leg.
- Bend the standing leg slightly.
- The toes should point naturally down as you raise your left foot.

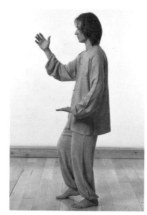

123 Put your right foot down on its toes in front of your left, and shift your weight onto it. Turn your body to the left, using the ball of your left toes as a pivot.

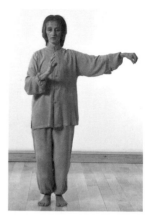

124 Raise your left hand to the side to shoulder height and make a left hooked hand.

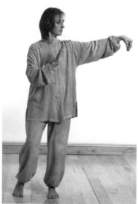

125 Your right hand, following the body turn, moves in an arc until it comes in front of your left shoulder with the fingers pointing up. Look at your left hand.

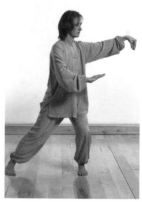

126 Bend your left knee, stretching your right leg to the side (to 4 o'clock). Extend your right hand along your inner right leg, palm facing forward.

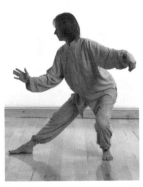

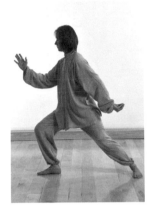

127 When your left leg is fully bent, turn the toes of your left foot out and straighten your right leg with the toes pointing forward.

128 Straighten your left leg and bend the right. Shift your weight to your right foot. Extend your right hand forward and drop the left behind, fingers bent.

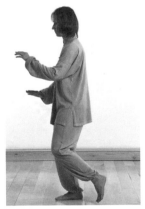

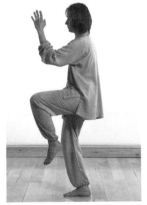

129 Begin to raise your left foot until your thigh is parallel to the floor.

130 Open your left hand and swing it up, until your elbow is above your left knee, fingers pointing up. Lower your right hand to your hip, palm down.

141

Step 18: Fair Lady Works Shuttles

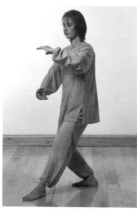 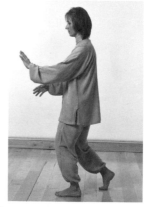

131 Turn to the left (to 1 o'clock). Put your left foot down, toes pointing out. Bend your knees. Make a hold-ball gesture with the left hand on top.

132 Shift your weight to your left foot, and move your right foot, on its toes, next to your left foot. Look at the left forearm.

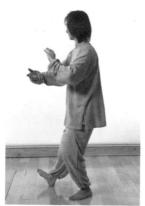

133 Sit back on your left foot and take a step with your right foot (to 4 o'clock).

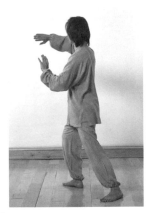

134 Complete the right bow stance.

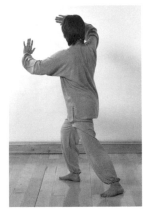

135 Move your right hand up to your right temple, palm up. Move your left hand down to the left side, and push it forward and up to nose level, palm forward.

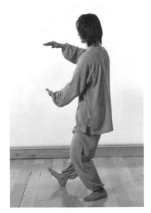

136 Turn slightly, shifting your weight back, with the toes of your right foot turned out. Make a hold-ball gesture with the right hand on top.

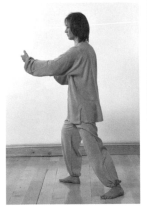

137 Shift your weight onto your right foot and place your left foot next to it with the heel raised and the toes on the floor.

143

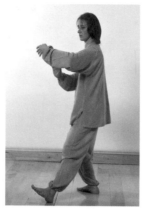

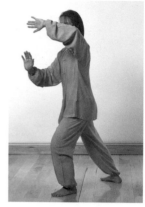

138 Turn to the left and take a step to 2 o'clock with the left foot, placing your heel down first.

139 Shift your weight onto your left foot to complete the left bow stance.

Points to Remember

• Do not lean forward when pushing your hands forward, or shrug your shoulders when raising your hands.

• Coordinate the movements of the hands with those of your waist and legs.

• The distance between your heels in the bow steps is about 30 cm (12 in).

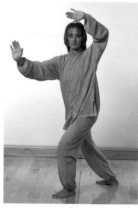

140 Move your left hand up to your left temple, palm up. Move your right hand down to the right and push it forward and up to nose level, palm forward.

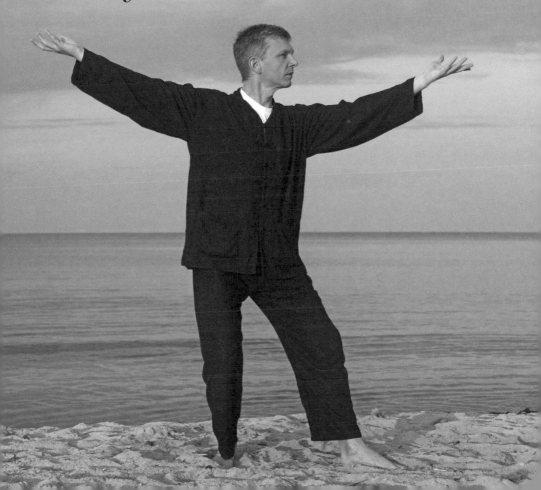

'*Your attention resides in your Tan Tien throughout The Form so that your movements issue from your centre and radiate out to your head and limbs.*'

Step19: Needle at Sea Bottom

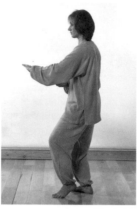 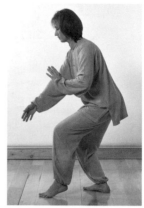

141 Take half a step forward with your right foot. Shift your weight onto your right foot as your left foot moves forward to form a left empty stance. Turn your body to the right (to 4 o'clock).

142 Lower your right hand, then raise it to your right ear. Turning to 3 o'clock, thrust it down in front of you, palm in, fingers down. Make an arc with your left hand, forward and down to your left hip, palm down, fingers forward.

Points to Remember

- In the empty stance, the toes come down on the floor first.
- Do not lean too far forward.
- Keep your head erect and your seat tucked in.

'Remember when moving, there is no place that does not move.'

Wu Yuxiang

Step 20: Fan Penetrates Back

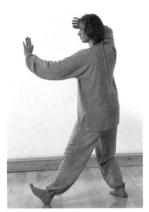 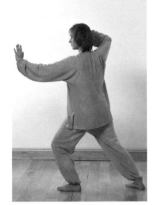

143 Turn slightly to the right. Make a left bow step forward. At the same time, raise your right arm with your elbow bent until your right hand stops just above your right temple.

144 Complete the bow stance. Tilt the palm up with the thumb pointing down. Raise your left hand slightly and push it forward at nose level, palm facing forward. Look at your left hand (to 2 o'clock). The distance between your heels should be about 10 cm (4 in).

Points to Remember

- Keep your upper body erect, and relax your waist and hips as well as the muscles in your back.
- Coordinate the movement of your left leg with that of your left arm.

147

Step 21: Turn, Deflect Downward, Parry and Punch

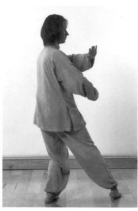

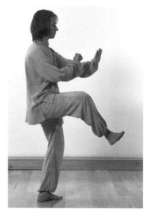

145 Shift your weight to your right foot, turn right, and shift it back to your left. Turn to face 6 o'clock, circle your right hand to the right and down. Make a fist, move it to your left side, knuckles up. Raise your left arm above your head, palm up.

146 Turn your body to the right. Thrust your right fist up and forward in front of your chest, knuckles down. Lower your left hand to the side of your left hip, palm turned downward and fingers forward. At the same time, draw back your right foot and, without stopping or allowing it to touch the floor, take a step to 10 o'clock with the toes turned out.

Points to Remember

- Clench your right fist loosely.
- While pulling back your fist, your forearm is first turned in, then out.
- While the fist strikes forward, your right shoulder follows the movement and extends slightly forward.
- Hold your shoulder and elbows down.

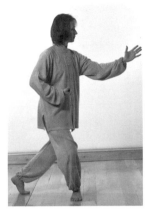

147 Shift your weight to your right foot. Move your left hand up and forward from the left in a circular movement, palm down. Pull the right fist in to the waist, knuckles down.

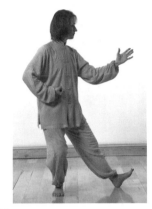

148 Take a step forward with your left foot. Look at your left hand (to 9 o'clock).

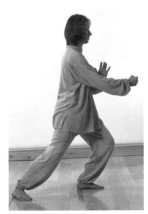

149 Strike forward with your right fist at chest height with the back of the hand facing out. Pull your left hand back to the side of the right forearm.

149

Step 22: Withdraw and Push

Points to Remember

- Do not lean backward when sitting back.
- Keep your buttocks in.
- Relax your shoulders and turn your elbows slightly out as you pull back your arms as your body moves.
- Do not pull your arms back straight.
- Your hands should be shoulder-width apart.

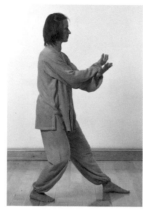

150 Stretch your left hand under your right wrist. Turn both palms up, separate your hands until they are shoulder-width apart and pull them back.

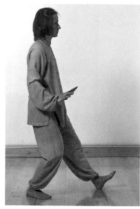

151 Sit back onto your right foot, with the toes of your left foot raised. Pull your hands down to your waist.

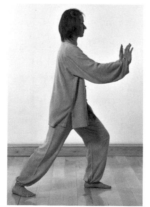

152 Complete the left bow step and push your palms forward and up to shoulder height, palms facing out. Look between your hands (to 9 o'clock).

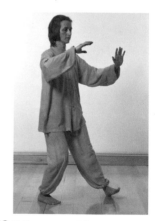

153 Shift your weight onto your right foot. Turn to the right and pivot on your left toes.

Step 23: Cross Hands

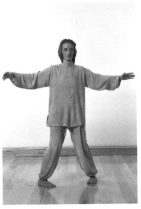

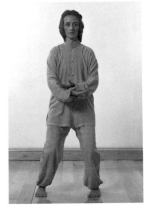

154 Circle your hands to shoulder height, palms forward, elbows slightly bent. Turn your right toes out, and shift your weight onto your right foot.

155 Shift your weight to your left foot, and turn your right toes in. Bring the right foot toward your left foot, to stand in shoulder-width stance.

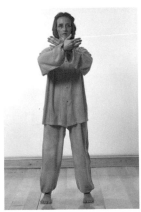

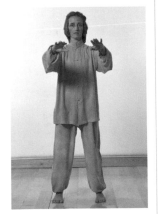

156 Straighten your legs. Cross both hands in front of you and raise them, wrists at shoulder height, right hand on the outside, both palms facing in.

157 You are facing 12 o'clock. Separate your hands, keeping them at shoulder height. Look forward. You are now in the starting position of The Form.

Points to Remember

- Do not lean forward when separating or crossing your hands.
- When making the parallel stance, keep your body naturally straight, with your head suspended and your chin tucked slightly inward.
- Keep your arms rounded in a comfortable position, with your shoulders and elbows down.

151

Step 24: Closing Form

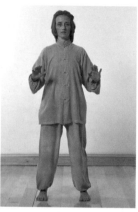 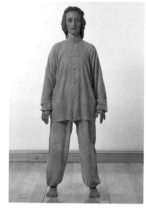

158 Turn your palms forward and down while lowering both arms gradually to the side of your hips.

159 Keep your entire body relaxed and draw a deep, prolonged breath as you lower both hands to your sides. Continue to look straight ahead to 12 o'clock. You may now commence another round of The Form.

'The twenty-four steps of The Form flow into one another to become one seamless movement, performed at a constant speed.'

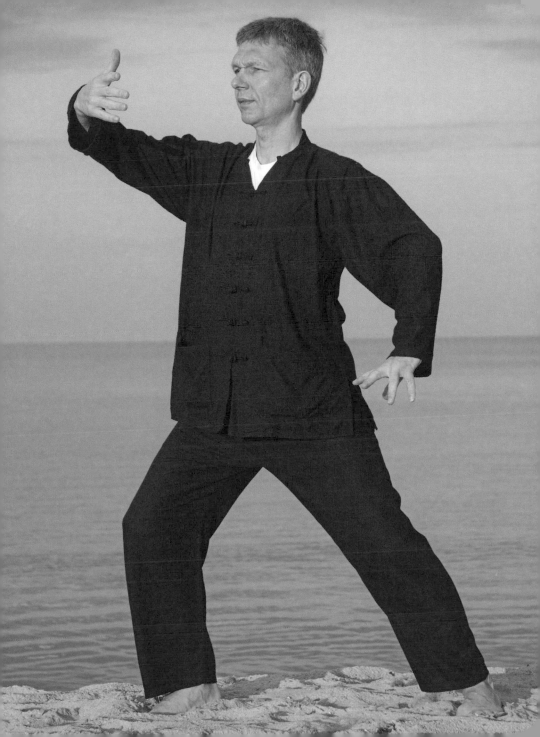

Two-person Practice
Strength Through Softness

The Tai Chi Form has its roots in the Chinese martial arts tradition, in which testing yourself against an opponent is the best way of discovering how far you have progressed. But unlike the 'hard' styles of kung-fu, in which the aim is to knock down an opponent with the sheer brute strength of a punch or kick, Tai Chi uses softness as its main weapon; it yields to pressure and deflects blows, and turns their power against the aggressor. This principle is epitomised by a saying of the great Tai Chi teacher, Wang Zongyue (1736–1795): 'From the sentence "a force of four ounces deflects a thousand pounds", we know that the technique is not accomplished through strength.'

Two-person practice (also known as push-hands) is not intended to show how strong you have become, but to reveal the exact opposite: to see if you are able to yield completely to your partner's movements, never presenting a square inch of hardness on your body. In this way, you learn to 'read' your partner's movements.

In the early stages of Tai Chi study, two-person practice is an invaluable help in discovering any faults in the Tai Chi principles you are learning in The Form. Are your feet properly rooted to the ground? Does your waist turn freely? Are your shoulders and arms rounded and relaxed? If your feet are unbalanced, then your partner can easily push you over; and if your waist or arms are stiff, he or she can use them as levers to topple you.

Single Circling Hands

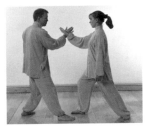

1 Stand with your feet shoulder-width apart, right foot forward and left foot turned out. Bend your knees. Your partner mirrors your stance, 1 m (3 ft) away.

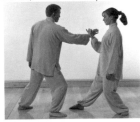

3 Keep both feet flat on the floor. When you move forward, do not push against your partner's hand, merely follow him as he retreats.

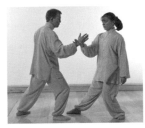

5 Your partner follows with the same movement. Keep your knees bent and focus your mind in your body's centre of gravity, your *dantian*.

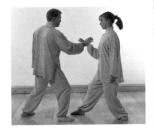

2 Raise your right arm in front of your chest. Make contact with your partner's raised arm lightly with the back of your hand, near his or her wrist.

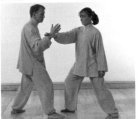

4 Once you and your partner are comfortable with the forward and backward motion, turn your waist and make a circular motion with your hand.

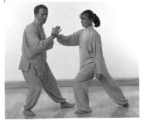

6 After 10–15 minutes, repeat with your left foot forward, circling with your right arm.

Double Circling Hands

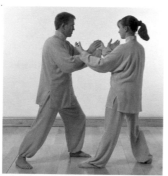

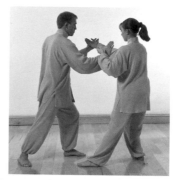

1 Once you and your partner are moving freely in the one-handed practice, you can attempt the two-handed version shown here. In the same stance as the one-handed form, link both hands lightly near the wrists.

2 Shift your weight from your front to rear foot. Add the rotation of your waist as before.

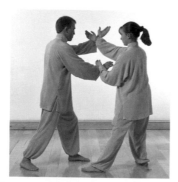

3 Make a circular motion with your hands, extending your arms as you lean forward, and withdrawing them as you lean back.

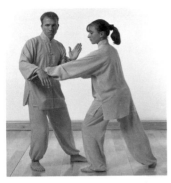

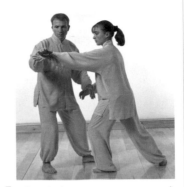

4 You may, at this stage, wish to challenge your partner to try to 'uproot' you. This does not mean he or she has to pick you up and throw you to the floor, but to try to find a place of hardness in your body to get you off balance. As you practise, keep your mind centred in your *Tan Tien*.

5 When it is your turn to extend, imagine your qi travelling up along your spine, to your shoulders, along your arms, and out of your hands. Practise both the one- and two-handed two-person exercises with your eyes closed to enable you to use your sense of touch only to gauge your partner's movements.

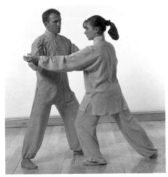

6 If you try to push your partner with brute force, he or she will make use of the hardness you manifest to push or pull you off balance. After 10–15 minutes, repeat with the opposite leg forward.

157

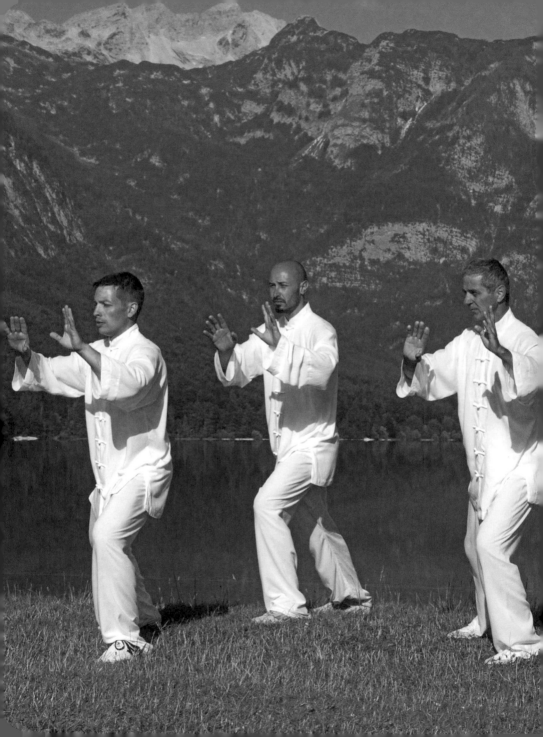

The Form at a Glance

Once you have learned The Form, you can practise it with greater fluidity, maintaining a constant pace throughout. The following pages present the entire sequence at a glance so that you can follow without the interruption of turning too many pages.

Twenty-four-step Tai Chi

The detailed instructions in the previous chapter break down each step of The Form so you can move from one step to the next in single fluid movements. Once you have learned the steps, you can use this chapter as a quick reference to speed up your Tai Chi practice, and to commit the moves to memory.

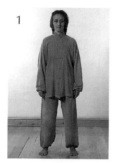
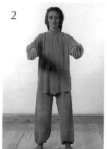
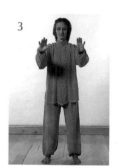

Step 1: Commencing Form

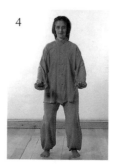
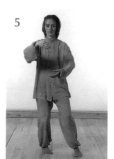
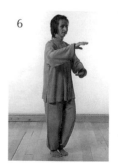

Step 2: Part Wild Horse Mane on Both Sides

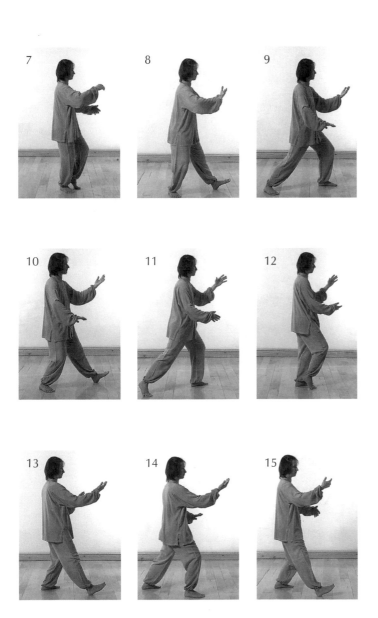

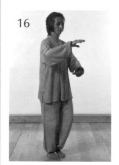

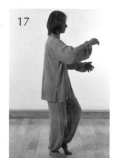

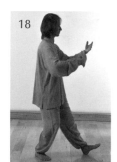

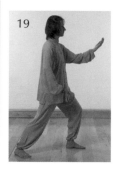

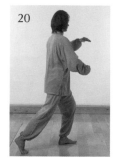

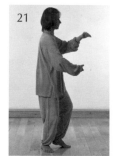

Step 3: White Crane Spreads its Wings

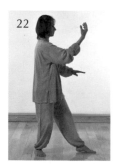

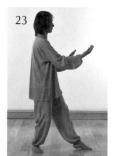

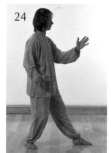

Step 4: Brush Knee and Twist Step on Both Sides

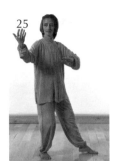

25

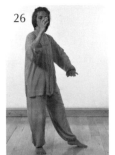

26

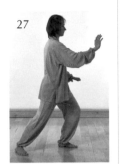

27

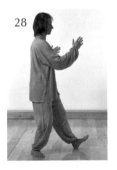

28

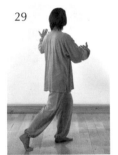

29

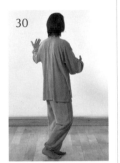

30

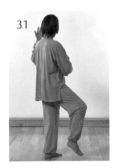

31

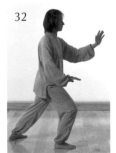

32

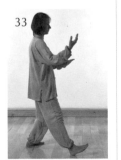

33

163

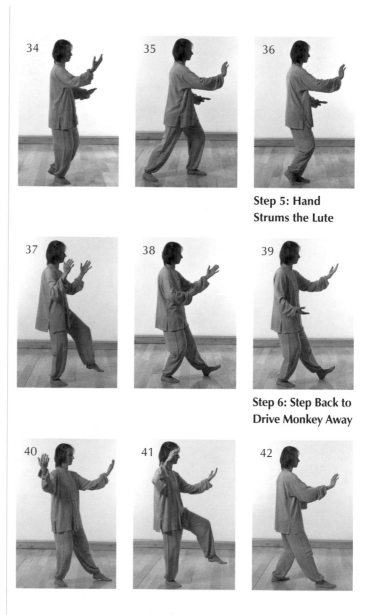

Step 5: Hand Strums the Lute

Step 6: Step Back to Drive Monkey Away

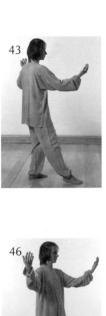

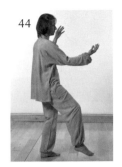

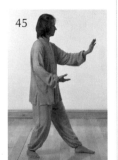

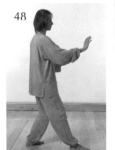

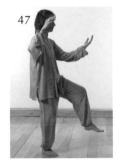

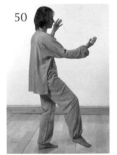

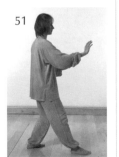

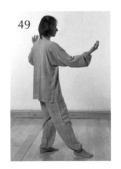

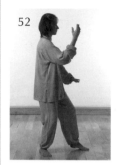
52

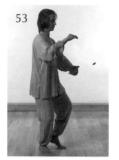
53

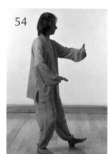
54

Step 7: Grasp the Bird's Tail – Left Style

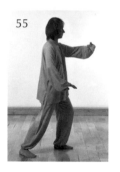
55

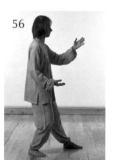
56

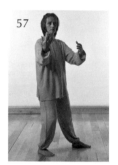
57

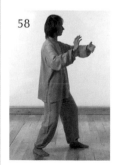
58

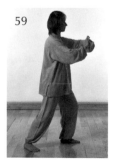
59

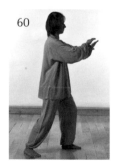
60

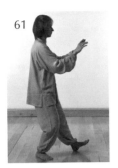

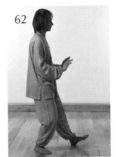

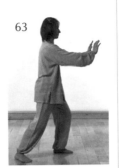

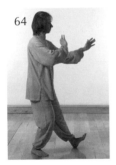

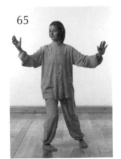

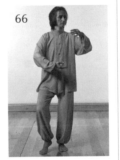

Step 8: Grasp the Bird's Tail – Right Style

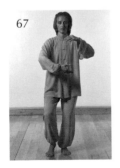

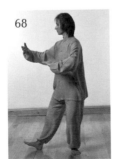

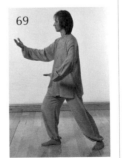

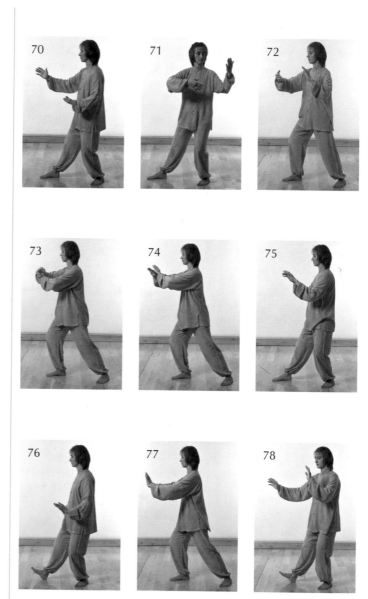

Step 9: Single Whip

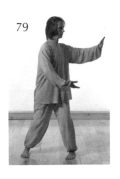

79

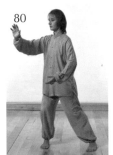

80

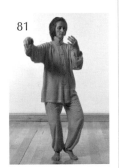

81

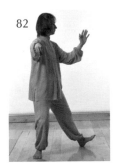

82

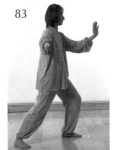

83

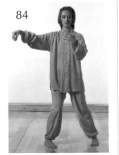

84

**Step 10:Wave
Hands Like Clouds**

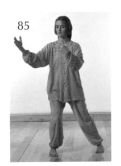

85

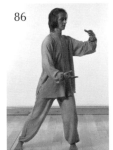

86

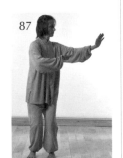

87

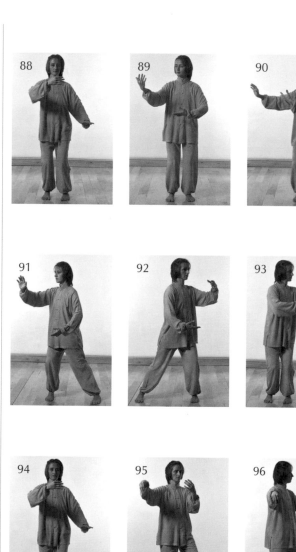

Step 11: Single Whip

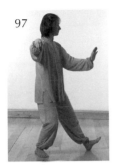
97

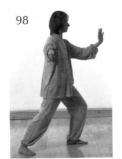
98

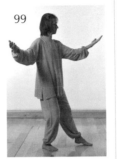
99

Step 12: High Pat on Horse

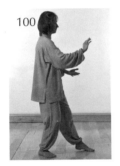
100

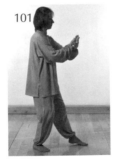
101

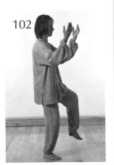
102

Step 13: Kick with Right Heel

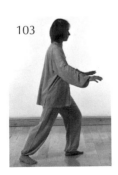
103

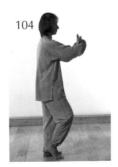
104

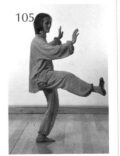
105

171

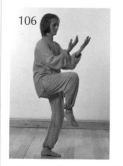

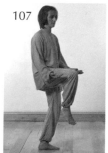

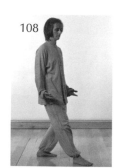

Step 14: Strike with Both Fists

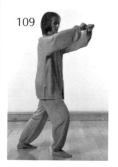

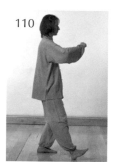

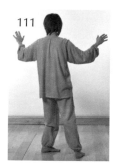

Step 15: Turn and Kick with Left Heel

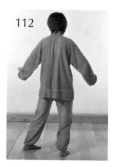

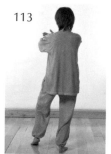

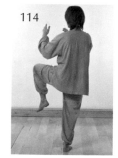

172

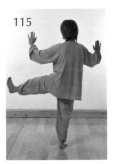

115

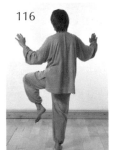

116

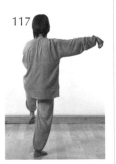

117

Step 16: Squat Down and Stand on One Leg – Left Style

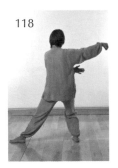

118

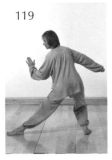

119

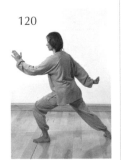

120

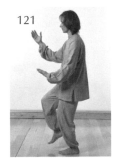

121

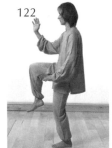

122

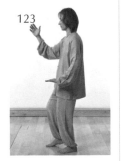

123

Step 17: Squat Down and Stand on One Leg – Right Style

173

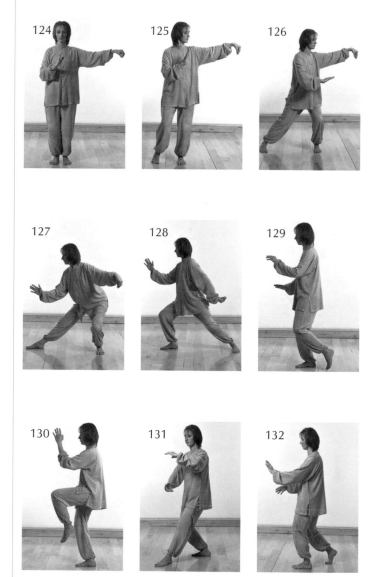

Step 18: Fair Lady Works the Shuttles

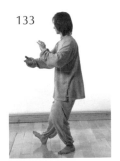

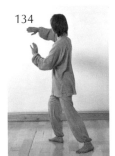

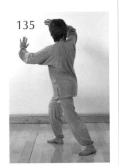

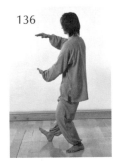

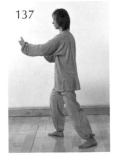

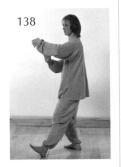

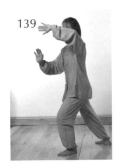

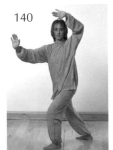

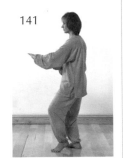

**Step 19: Needle at
Sea Bottom**

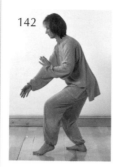 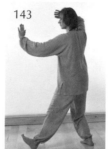 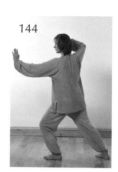

Step 20: Fan Penetrates Back

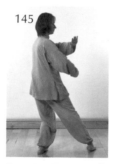 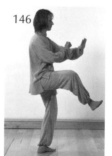 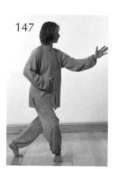

Step 21: Turn, Deflect Downward, Parry and Punch

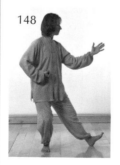 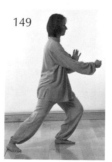 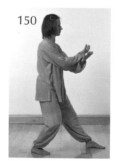

Step 22: Withdraw and Push

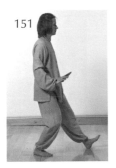

151

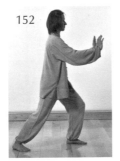

152

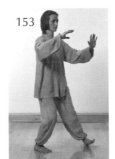

153

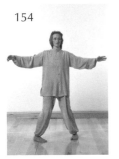

154

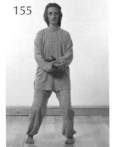

155

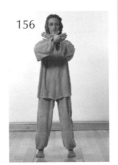

156

Step 23: Cross Hands

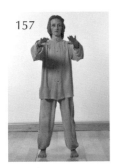

157

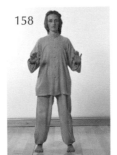

158

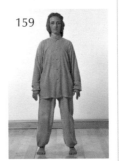

159

Step 24: Closing Form

177

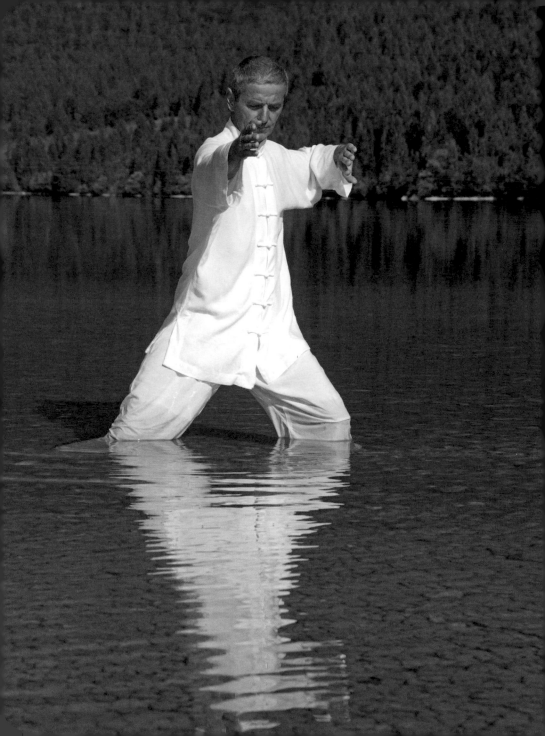

Specific Applications

While the main goal of practising Tai Chi is to unite mind, body and spirit, there are numerous other benefits to be gained by performing the movements on a regular basis.

Specific Applications

Most people take their bodies for granted. As a rule, it is only when their attention is involuntarily drawn to it, through injury, illness or, in the case of women, pregnancy, that they focus on their bodies. In Chinese eyes, this is a typical Western attitude. A Chinese physician is someone who helps a person to stay well; in the West, people resort to a doctor to make them better. If you think about it, the Chinese approach is the more sensible one.

Tai Chi is part of the Chinese system of keeping well. The following section describes some of the benefits that the art bestows on its students. Some of them are curative and some preventative. They are based on knowledge derived from traditional Chinese medicine, and the application of that knowledge over several centuries to the specific movements of Tai Chi. The benefits of Tai Chi are interdependent. You cannot have one without the other. As you read more about the subject, and then as you train and study, this will become apparent.

Head and Neck

The relationship between head and neck can be vastly improved through the correct performance of Tai Chi. The head is 'carried' by the neck. See pages 183–185.

Head and Spine

The head should be a 'free' extension of the spine. This means that it can work in concert with the vertebrae, but also independently. See pages 186–187.

Circulation

Tai Chi is the best form of exercise for improving the circulation of energy and Chi. After some time you should feel the benefits in the hands and feet. See pages 188 189.

Muscle Tone

The tone of the muscles should be neither too Yin nor too Yang; that is, optimum, the best there is. Prolonged training can produce this happy state of affairs. See pages 190–191.

Correct Joint Use

As you perform Tai Chi you inevitably learn the correct use of most of the joints of the body. You may even begin to wonder why you never discovered it for yourself. See page 192.

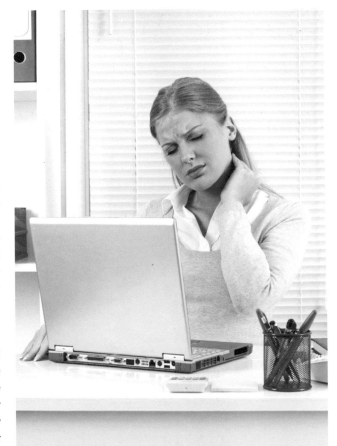

Digestion

Tai Chi is meant to relax the body, uniformly, and to distribute the energy, uniformly. This soothes the body and helps to promote better digestion. See page 193.

Balance

Correct Tai Chi training should improve your balance and banish the deep-seated fear of falling. You begin to feel solidly rooted on the earth. See pages 194–195.

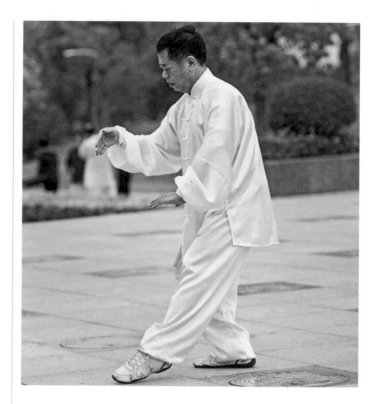

Stress

Stress is all about trying to do something at the wrong time. To do Tai Chi well you have to live in the present moment, where there is no stress. See pages 196–197.

Other Benefits

Tai Chi can produce a previously unknown feeling of calm, associated with the peace of natural scenes, softly swaying grasses and placid lakes. See page 198.

Older People

No one has yet discovered a cure for old age, but Tai Chi can defeat the growing immobility which afflicts elderly people. Can millions of Chinese be wrong? See page 199.

Head and Neck

The neck is a very important area of the body. Problems with the vertebrae, muscles and nerves in this area can cause stiffness, pain, headaches and tension.

Joints

Joints not only enable us to move the way we do, but also facilitate the flow of blood and Chi. However, incorrectly used, they can impede this flow. If you lift your chin high, you can feel the bones and muscles at the back of the neck contract and close together. You don't need any medical knowledge to realise that this position blocks the flow of energy through the region. This is an extreme example since you cannot help but be aware of the tension. However, most people have a lot of unrecognised and unnecessary tension in this part of the body, which affects their feeling of well-being.

Below Balance your head and look life quietly in the face ...

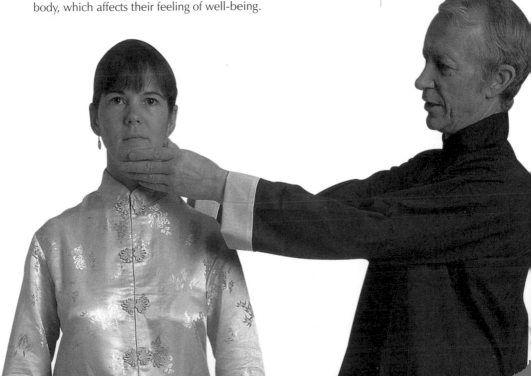

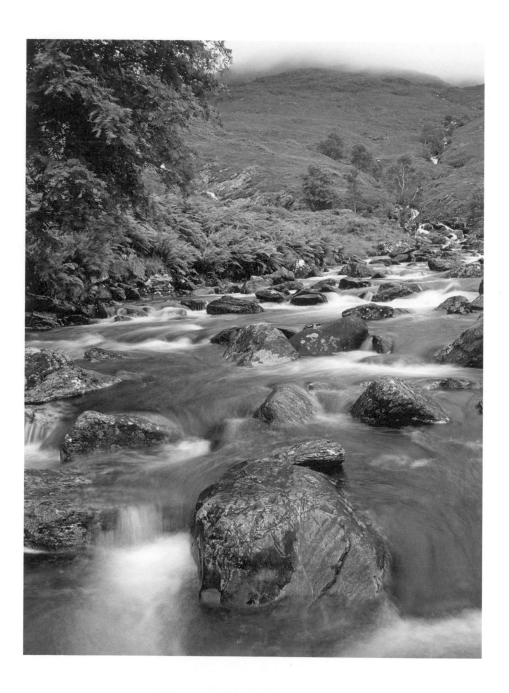

Chi and Energy

In Chinese terms, this blocking of energy means that the Chi and the blood are not able to flow naturally from the body, into the head, and back down into the body. At the point where the tension begins there is an excess (stagnancy) of Chi, and at the point where the tension ends there is a deficit of Chi. Treating this pattern of excess–stagnancy–deficiency is a basic principle of traditional Chinese medicine.

Breathing

This new relationship between the head and the neck is not easy to attain. But if you practise Tai Chi regularly, you will reach it. One of the benefits, in addition to the flow of energy, is that breathing will tend to deepen. If the muscles of the neck region are too contracted, the chest cannot rise and fall as well as it might, and breathing action will be restricted.

As the head begins to float up, the chest will sink, the ribcage becomes free and the abdomen begins to take part in breathing. When you start experiencing this new, deeper breathing, which should come naturally and not be forced in any way, you will begin to realise that 'breath is life' and that breathing correctly increases your energy, reduces stress and helps you sleep.

Once you know some of The Form (see pages 98–157) well, it is a good idea to go through it specifically focusing on letting your head 'float' up, while giving less attention to the other movements. To help yourself in this direction, try to relax your forehead and orbits of the eyes. Release your jaw and let the chin drop down a little.

A word of warning: it is not possible to isolate one part of the body from another, and what is said in this section should be combined with the information and advice given elsewhere in the book.

A Relaxed Approach

Tai Chi has its own healing formula of relaxation, gentle movement and working toward the posture of 'head suspended from above as if by a single hair'. The sensation to aim for when doing The Form is one of the head being lightly carried on the top of the spine; the head floating up, while the rest of the body sinks down.

185

Head and Spine

Western, as well as Chinese, healers have recognised the importance of the occiput to health. This is the place where the skull rests on the top of the spine. Bad posture means that the neck muscles are unnecessarily contracted, impeding the flow of the Chi and causing tension and potential back problems as well as shallow breathing.

Tai Chi places great emphasis on correct posture. The Tai Chi maxim states that the head should be suspended above the vertebrae as if held by a single hair. Although this floating posture is not literally physically attainable, the maxim describes how your head and neck should feel when you are practising Tai Chi correctly.

Right Do not crunch your head on to your neck.

Posture

Children naturally have good posture, but bad habits form as we grow older. Often a particular way of standing or holding the head becomes a habit, placing strain on the vertebrae and muscles and causing stress and potential damage. The head becomes jammed down onto the spine like a tight hat, bent back or hung forward. It is rarely in the optimum position the Chinese maxim describes.

Chi

The saying that the Chi must go down implies that it must also, at some stage, go up. According to Tai Chi theory, the Chi descends down the front of the body along one of the major channels and ascends up the spine, over the top of the head, and down again. Congestion in the occipital region hinders this flow.

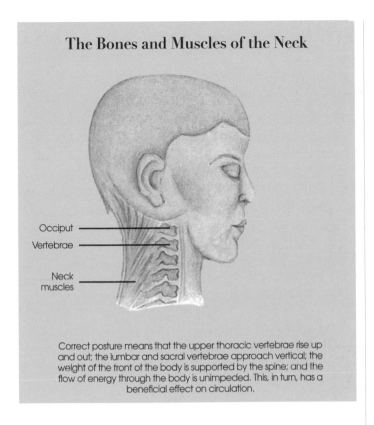

The Bones and Muscles of the Neck

Occiput

Vertebrae

Neck
muscles

Correct posture means that the upper thoracic vertebrae rise up and out; the lumbar and sacral vertebrae approach vertical; the weight of the front of the body is supported by the spine; and the flow of energy through the body is unimpeded. This, in turn, has a beneficial effect on circulation.

Tai Chi training, with its emphasis on letting the head float up naturally, focuses on the vertebrae, training the spine to fall into a more natural position and bringing the entire body into alignment.

'Tai Chi Chuan is like a great river rolling on unceasingly.'

ZHANG SANFENG

187

Circulation

Everyone knows that good blood circulation is important: oxygen, nutrients, carbon dioxide and waste products depend on it. Closely allied with circulation are heart rate and breathing. Traditional Chinese Medicine carries this a stage further and adds that these functions of the body depend on an optimum supply of Chi – neither too much, nor too little. The Chi helps the circulation of the blood.

L ifestyle, of course, strongly influences circulation. A fixed routine, for instance, results in an established and repetitive circulation. In contrast, a hectic pace of life means that the restorative part of the nervous system has little chance to operate. In both cases, traditional Chinese medicine sees Tai Chi as a means of bringing the circulation back into balance.

With its slow, even pace, Tai Chi stimulates the restorative powers of the body when you are neither asleep nor resting. From one point of view the movements are like a slow self-massage without hands! When the muscles are trained to relax, they move easily from relaxation to tension and back again, pumping the blood and lymphatic fluid back toward the heart and lungs in a steady, even way.

In time, breathing will deepen as you learn to use the diaphragm muscles to greater effect, thus improving the intake of oxygen. Your heart rate will become more regular and even slower. And you will notice that the recovery back to your normal heart rate after exercise will take less time.

Once again, you can see that everything in Tai Chi is linked together and that it is impossible to isolate any one element.

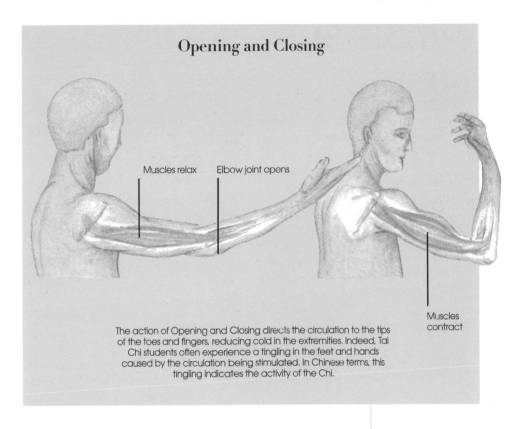

Opening and Closing

Muscles relax

Elbow joint opens

Muscles contract

The action of Opening and Closing directs the circulation to the tips of the toes and fingers, reducing cold in the extremities. Indeed, Tai Chi students often experience a tingling in the feet and hands caused by the circulation being stimulated. In Chinese terms, this tingling indicates the activity of the Chi.

'If the body is clumsy, then in advancing or retreating, it cannot be free.'

LI YIYU

189

Muscle Tone

As far as health is concerned, it is preferable to have what is called good muscle tone rather than strength. Muscles can be very soft and flabby, Yin, or hard as iron, Yang. Good tone is somewhere in between these two extremes: a condition in which the very small elements that make up a muscle are at their 'happiest'. In this condition they are best able to relax more or to tense more, whatever is required.

Tai Chi cultivates smoothness of action and this is what muscles in general like. Muscles work in a two-way fashion. When the biceps flex in the upper arm, the triceps extend in the upper arm. The biceps are the agonist muscles when they cause the arm to bend, and the triceps are the antagonist muscles. When the arm is straightened, the two muscle groups reverse their roles. Without an antagonist muscle the action of the agonist muscle could not be controlled.

So smoothness of action means that the relation between the two muscle groups is optimum. In an ideal situation all the muscle groups of the body would synchronise harmoniously, and the resulting benefit to the body would be incredible.

When a muscle stretches, there is a built-in tendency for it to want to go back in the opposite direction. This is called a stretch reflex. Interestingly, it is in harmony with a fundamental principle of the Yin-Yang theory. This propounds that when any phenomenon reaches its maximum Yin or Yang condition, it naturally begins to move in the opposite direction.

When moving in haste there is no time to think about your muscles or about the effect the movement may have on them. In Tai Chi there is ample time to get in tune with your body and to listen to what it is telling you.

Learning The Form is like learning to play a musical instrument – your first efforts will be clumsy and uncoordinated. However, once you have acquired skill, you are able to produce fine differences in tone and volume. Likewise, once you know the basic movements of The Form, you will be able to fine-tune your actions so that muscle tone, smoothness of movement, awareness of flex, reflex and feedback all combine harmoniously. This is an ideal condition for the flow of Chi.

If you make Tai Chi part of your daily life, you will find that concentrating on this harmony of movement will firm up your muscles and improve your level of fitness.

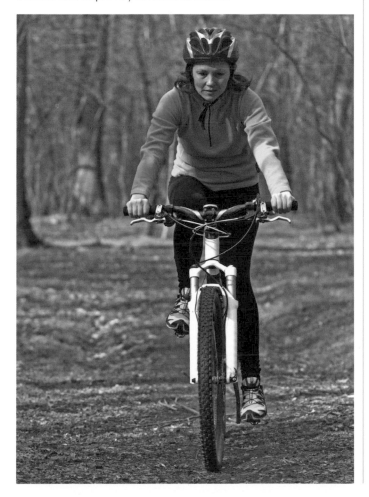

Left Other forms of gentle exercise, such as cycling, walking and swimming, can be very beneficial for muscle tone.

191

Correct Joint Use

Good muscle tone can work in harmony with correct use of the joints. Because we are not in general as closely in touch with our physical activity as animals are, we are not nearly as aware of what they are doing. We often misuse our joints, compelling them to move in ways for which they are not designed.

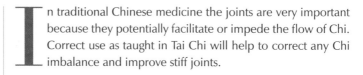

I n traditional Chinese medicine the joints are very important because they potentially facilitate or impede the flow of Chi. Correct use as taught in Tai Chi will help to correct any Chi imbalance and improve stiff joints.

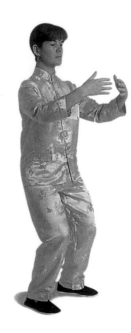

Knee and Ankle Joints

The knee and ankle joints are ideal for illustrating joint use. Both are hinge joints, working more or less like the hinge of a door. This means that when you bend your knee and ankle, the knee should move forward over the foot. If you stand up and look down at your feet, then bend your knees, you should lose sight of your feet. If your knees move outward or your lower leg falls inward, this is wrong and places a strain on the joints. In Tai Chi the knee should not extend beyond the toes.

Elbow Joint

The elbow is also a hinge joint but at the top of the forearm there is another joint which enables it to rotate. In Tai Chi both of these joints are fully used, and the maxim that the elbows should be down is incorporated into The Form. This means that the shoulder joints are not in a constant state of tension holding the whole arm up. There is less strain on the chest, which leads to greater ease of breathing.

Wrist Joint

The wrist joint can act like a hinge, rotate, and turn from side to side. If you go more deeply into Tai Chi, you will learn how to use the wrist joint in combination with the extending and contracting of the palm.

Digestion

Traditional Chinese medicine says that human beings contain a number of vital energies and substances. These are Shen (spirit), Jing (vital energy released), Chi (intrinsic energy), blood (blood and the functions of blood) and fluids (sweat, urine). Shen is the finest, fluids are the coarsest.

These five are linked together in an ascending chain. Shen is the highest product. If there is anything wrong with any of them, then the whole chain is disrupted. This is true in the eyes of Western medicine too. If there is something wrong with any organ of digestion and elimination, then the whole body will be affected.

Beginning with the mouth, it is traditional in Tai Chi to keep the·tip of the tongue lightly in contact with the roof of the mouth behind the teeth. This stimulates the flow of saliva, which is swallowed slowly. The calm feeling accompanying Tai Chi helps to 'comfort' the stomach and other organs, all of which contributes to good digestion.

The regular breathing and slow, even body movement 'massage' the organs and help to regulate their activity. And the ordered Chi flow contributes the energy necessary for their good functioning.

The liver is regarded as a very important organ in traditional Chinese medicine. Certain movements of The Form – for instance, Single Whip (page 129), done with the left arm leading – are said to be particularly beneficial to the liver. It is not advisable, except under the guidance of a knowledgeable teacher, to perform single repetitions of a movement to attain a particular benefit. Step Back To Drive Monkey Away (page 113) is said to benefit the kidney function, especially in women.

Finally, Tai Chi can be very beneficial for constipation. The overall feeling generated by The Form induces the large intestine to return to normal and the movements themselves seem to aid peristalsis.

Balance

It is not an exaggeration to say that many people are, to a large extent, cut off from the sensations of abdomen and legs. They do not experience that they are on the earth – quite literally. Small wonder then that if they feel they may lose their balance and fall, they are afraid. They are not sure where they may go if they fall. They are out of touch with what holds them up, their legs.

Tai Chi is sometimes called 'mediation in movement'. The posture of seated meditation focuses energy in the lower abdomen. The ideal centre of gravity in a standing human being is in the lower abdomen. In Tai Chi, the cultivation of the lower abdomen, its strength and fullness, shows that people in the East have realised for centuries that their health and power reside much lower down than is believed in the West. The posture of seated meditation focuses the energy in this region.

Training

Tai Chi training brings people down to earth. Letting the Chi go down, sinking the elbows, bending the knees, placing the feet correctly, and the rest of the Tai Chi maxims all combine to replace the Western emphasis on the upper body with a new one. This is based on simple observation. Gravity keeps human beings glued on the earth, and the nearest contact with gravity is your feet! Tai Chi says that people should build upward from their feet, not downward from their brains. This really makes sense! To carry this sense of gravity a stage further, imagine yourself to be a tree and that your feet are roots. When a tree is blown by the wind, it bends, yields, but remains in place. This sense of being rooted takes time to acquire. During the first few months of learning Tai Chi, you will need to absorb some of the basic principles of balance mentioned above.

As these principles begin to penetrate your rendering of The Form, you will one day feel, perhaps briefly, that the upper part of your body seems 'empty', Yin, and the lower part seems 'full',

Yang. When this happens, it is like entering a different world. You have the impression that suddenly you fit into things, into Nature, and that your usual state of mind is one of unnecessary struggling.

If you go on to study Push Hands, training with a partner, you will see that this new condition is an ideal one. When your partner pushes you, your upper body can yield. You do not fall because your lower body is anchored to the ground. Even if you take steps forward or backward, when your feet land, they root to the ground.

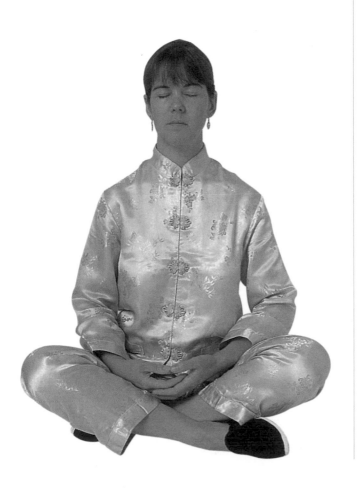

Stress

Stress can be seen partly as a result of over-reaction to stimuli of daily life, and partly as a result of the unprecedented pace of modern life. If you are being constantly stimulated by telephone, email, letters, people, chores and work pressures, your body and brain do not have time to relax, even if they want to.

Tai Chi, like yoga, is more than just a series of exercises; the body is inextricably linked with the mind. Practising The Form requires concentration, pushing worries and unrelated thoughts from the mind. Increased physical well-being brings with it a more relaxed state of mind. In time, you will be able to recreate this feeling of relaxation when you are going about your daily life.

Stress is an attempt to cope with seemingly impossible situations. When you are immersed in them, they seem insoluble. If you can move out of them, you gain a different perspective. Tai Chi is a way of moving out of one situation and into another. The advantage is that you do not have to travel very far – just to your Tai Chi place. The whole focus of your attention moves toward the fundamental things of your life itself. The preoccupations of your mind and emotions become secondary.

If you train regularly at Tai Chi, you have to slow down. Tai Chi demands it. If possible, do your Tai Chi in a natural setting. If this is not possible, find somewhere secluded, at the last resort your bedroom. Train in the same place. This will build up good associations. The place will become a Tai Chi place for you, and when you go there, you will leave behind the demands of life. So much of stress centres around an apparent disorder. You struggle to reach some sense of order in a complex of perpetual disorder. In Tai Chi you are taught a natural order, and you try to become one with it. As you gradually succeed, through diligent training and study, you may begin to see the disorder of daily life differently. You may discover that it is not ultimately necessary to be swept away by it. The memory of your Tai Chi times can come back to you, reminding you that a different condition is very close at hand.

Meditation in Movement

The human brain displays at least five types of wave: delta – in deep sleep; theta – in light sleep; alpha – calm waking state; beta – active/ stressed state; and gamma – fighting pitch. Zen monks' brainwave patterns have been measured during meditation. They move very easily into the alpha range and soon afterwards into the theta range. Experienced Tai Chi students can experience a similar change, which is one of the reasons why Tai Chi is sometimes described as 'meditation in movement'.

This experience, on a regular basis, can introduce a sense of calm into daily life. However, like most benefits, this does not happen without effort. When doing a simple household or office task, move with the same relaxation and care you bring to The Form. The act of paying attention in a quiet way to some physical activity can move the brain pattern into the alpha and possibly toward the theta. This does not mean that you fall asleep; if anything, you become more awake. Regular practice will make it easier to recreate this experience of calm in a variety of situations, helping you to take greater control over your emotions and, thus, of your life.

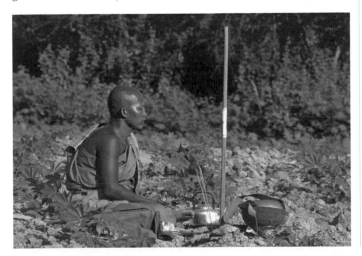

Left Tai Chi can be the dynamic expression of what monks experience in static meditation.

197

Other Benefits

Other benefits from Tai Chi are less easily classified, nor are they guaranteed. This is because they require a kind of feedback from the Tai Chi experiences themselves.

Right The symmetry of correct balance and posture.

Below Obvious down-the-middle symmetry.

For instance, on this page are illustrations of two types of symmetry. The second one is not geometrical, but depends on both the eye of the beholder and the posture itself. If a dancer or Tai Chi student takes a particular posture and holds it, he or she, or someone looking at him or her, may receive an impression which is very pleasing, aesthetically stimulating. If the performer or viewer thinks no more of the experience, then the benefit will be short lived. If, on the other hand, either of them reflect on it, and start to assume much better postures in daily life, with the benefits which come from that, then the Tai Chi training and daily life will exert a reciprocal influence and a perennially useful lesson will have been learned.

198

Older People

As people get older, their health and vitality tends to diminish. How quickly this happens depends on a number of things, but Tai Chi is traditionally regarded as a means of resisting this process.

That does not necessarily mean increasing the number of years of one's life, but rather maintaining youthfulness at a higher level than would otherwise have been the case.

After World War II the Chinese began investigating the benefits of Tai Chi for the elderly in a more scientific way. They carried out surveys of practitioners of a certain age, comparing them with non-practitioners. In one such project, people aged between fifty and eighty-nine were chosen. The findings showed that among Tai Chi students the cardiovascular level was much better, breathing was deeper and more efficient, the strength of the bones and use of the joints was markedly superior and metabolism in general was well maintained. Both groups were also asked to step up and down a bench some 40 cm (14 in) high and readings were taken of their respiratory and heart functioning. Again, in this set experiment, the Tai Chi group showed a much higher efficiency rate. Both blood pressure and arteriosclerosis were lower. Elasticity of lung tissue and relative movement of the ribcage (which fends off ossification of the rib cartilages) were higher in the Tai Chi group.

With age, people feel less inclined to take exercise, but the exercise of Tai Chi is gentle and slow. This means that little demand is made on the heart, and yet Tai Chi conducts the blood supply to and from the extremities of the body, indeed to all parts of the body, helping to prevent the build-up of waste products due to poor circulation. It is also likely that the mobility of joints and good blood supply that result from practising Tai Chi regularly, promotes a happier outlook and ample oxygen for the brain. If a person gradually loses the capacity to move, this is almost bound to affect his or her attitude to, and enjoyment of life.

Below Older people discover a new meaning to their lives through the practice of Tai Chi and Chi Kung.

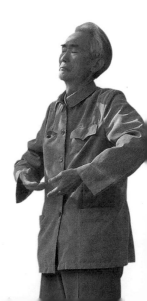

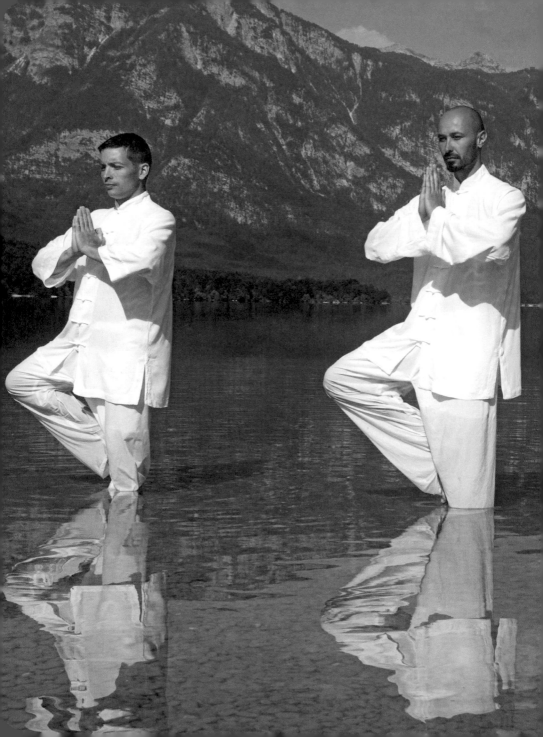

Meditation

Regular practice of meditation is integral to the way of life promoted by Tai Chi. It helps to focus the mind and is essential in uniting mind, body and spirit. As such, it is invaluable to your overall sense of well-being.

Introducing Meditation

We all have moments when we are so busy that we have to sit down and gather our thoughts for a few seconds. It is this same natural impulse that prompted our ancestors to begin meditating. Meditation is usually thought of as a spiritual exercise leading to enlightenment, but Tai Chi has discovered its practical dimension, which you can use, regardless of your religious beliefs, to improve your mental well-being. As a means of taking control of your thoughts and feelings, meditation is an ideal exercise to overcome the stress of modern-day life.

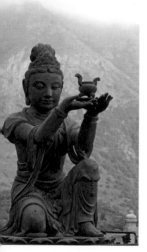

Above Buddhist zazen and Christian prayer lead to spiritual insight, but meditation also has a role to play in helping us find our mental equilibrium.

Stress is a mental condition that produces physical symptoms. Among the most common are sleeplessness, eating disorders and tiredness. We can deal with the symptoms of stress with medicines, but this is often at the cost of adding side effects, or if the symptoms are serious, drug dependence to our original problems. The only real cure for stress is to tackle its root causes, which are mental.

One-pointed Mind

In daily life, our attention always seems divided, confused, harassed. Yet we are not taught techniques that will help us detach ourselves from the worries and pressures of our home and professional lives. In its simplest form, meditation is making time for a moment of peace in our busy routine. To meditate, all you need to do is go to a tranquil place, close your eyes and clear your mind of all thoughts – good or bad. But to get the full benefits of meditation, you must not regard it as a passive activity like taking a catnap. Its ultimate aim is to give you the calmness and focus of the one-pointed mind that will enable you to control your thoughts and allow you to attain your full potential. In the beginning, you must be prepared to train your undisciplined mind as hard as you would train your unfit body.

Stillness in Motion

If you have attempted some of the exercises described in the earlier chapters of this book, you will know that Tai Chi is a unique combination of physical exercise and mental concentration, mediated and unified through the ancient Chinese concept of Chi. As such, it is the ideal antidote both to the physical symptoms of stress, as well as a way to deal with its mental causes. Stress becomes locked in our bodies in the form of tension in our muscles and joints, and unless it is released, it will damage us and lead to physical injury and illness.

All forms of movement, including dance, fitness training and sport, help us to deal with the physical symptoms of stress, because they allow us to release some of the tension locked in our bodies; however, as maintaining or restoring the holistic health of mind and body is not their primary function, their effectiveness remains limited. In fact, certain forms of conventional exercise, such as competitive sport and professional dance, which are mentally and physically very stressful, may make the problem worse.

Tai Chi employs a range of meditation techniques, some of which you will recognise from other traditions, such as hatha and tantric yoga, but it is in its joyous use of movement that it excels them all.

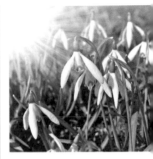

Above Opportunities to meditate are all around you: inspire yourself with the contemplation of the beauty and tranquility of nature.

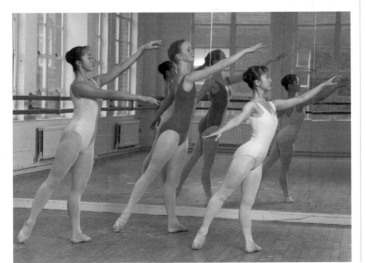

Left Mental stress becomes locked in our bodies and the easiest way to release it and prevent it from regaining its grip is through physical movement.

203

Moving Meditation

Life is movement, and the only true stillness is in death. Even when we are asleep, the continuous processes of life cause the tissues of our bodies to be renewed and repaired, and our minds to be refreshed through dreams.

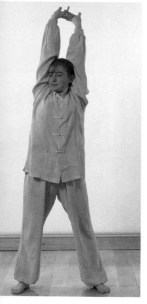

Above Link your hands, breathe in, and stretch your arms over your head, releasing the tension in your upper back and shoulders.

P eople often confuse meditation with trance, in which you give up control of your body, and sometimes of your conscious self, to another person or an external force, such as a mind-altering drug. The aim of meditation is the exact opposite: to give you complete control over your mind, and through your mind of your body.

All forms of meditation need a focus to still the mind, and later in this chapter, we will see how this can be achieved with breathing and visualisation techniques. But we will begin with Tai Chi's unique contribution to the world: moving meditation.

The Joyous Dance

Our bodies are not only designed to move, but also to enjoy movement. It is no accident that many of our most pleasurable and joyful activities – dancing, sport and making love – fully engage our minds, senses and bodies in harmonious movement. The Tai Chi Form itself is often described as a moving meditation, but its function is to combine body and mind to circulate and increase the Chi, in order to maintain and improve physical health. In moving meditation, the emphasis is reversed, and the motion of the body becomes the agent to centre the mind.

As such, you are freed from the constraints of following the exact and demanding movements and sequence of The Form. You can let your body experience the complete joyfulness of unfettered movement. Where The Form provides a discipline, moving meditation offers a joyous release of limitations – an invitation to explore and expand the boundaries of your physical being.

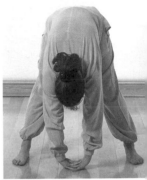

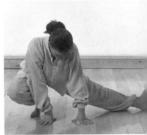

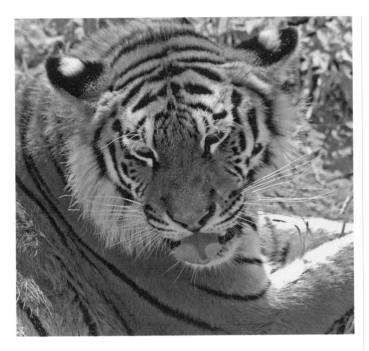

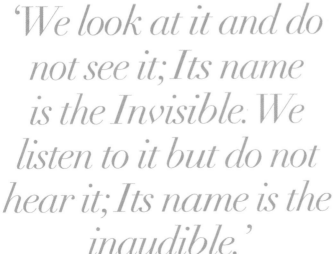

'We look at it and do
not see it; Its name
is the Invisible. We
listen to it but do not
hear it; Its name is the
inaudible.'

TAO THE CHING

Above Let your body move from position to position smoothly. Breathe in as you stretch up and out, and in as you pull down and in. Keep your mind focused in your Tan Tien, your body's centre of gravity.

205

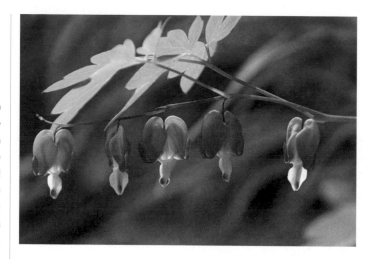

Below When performing the automatic motion exercise, the movements you will experience range from gentle swaying to dynamic jumps and arm swings.

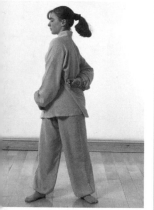

'To hold and fill a cup to overflowing is not as good as stopping.'

TAO THE CHING

Automatic Motion

This is a helpful exercise to those who have difficulty letting go of their bodies. Stand in shoulder-width stance, take a few deep breaths, and centre your attention in your Tan Tien. Tap your navel with your right hand and rub the top of your head with your left forefinger three times to start the flow of Chi. Perform six to nine repetitions of three of Chi Kung exercises. When you have finished, stand easy and imagine the Chi flowing down from your head and up from the soles of your feet. Allow your body to move at will, but remember your movements can become expansive and dynamic.

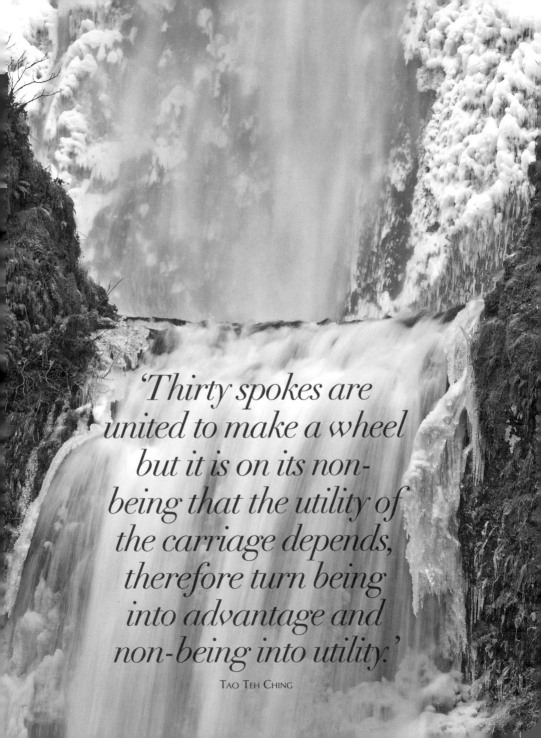

'Thirty spokes are
united to make a wheel
but it is on its non-
being that the utility of
the carriage depends,
therefore turn being
into advantage and
non-being into utility.'

TAO TEH CHING

Preparations for Moving Meditation

You do not need to study to attempt moving meditation; there are no complicated movements or sequences, no secret words or formulas to memorise. You stand like the first human, with only your mind, your body and the Universe around you.

As long as you are not exposed to extremes of heat or cold, you may prefer to perform this exercise clothed or naked, indoors or outdoors. All you require is a quiet space in which you feel completely comfortable, and that is large enough so that you take ten or so steps in any direction and swing your arms.

Stilling the Heart

Begin the meditation standing or kneeling in the centre of your chosen space, and close your eyes. Centre your mind in your Tan Tien. Breathe slowly and evenly, taking air in through your nose and expelling it through your mouth. Try and make the in and out breath last the same time, but without straining. As your breathing settles, notice how the beating of your heart slows to match it. Breathe for at least ten full breaths before moving on to the next stage.

Unlock the Gates

The next stage is to relax every muscle in your body and open every joint, so that the Chi can flow freely. Start with the muscles of your face and neck. Pay particular attention to the shoulders and upper back, where tension accumulates. Relax your arms, from the shoulders to the hands and down to the tiny muscles of the fingers. As you feel the tension

Some Gentle Cautions

In moving meditation, you may find your body moving in dynamic patterns. Should your movements become too rapid and expansive, immediately focus with your mind to regain control and slow yourself down. Remember that you are always in charge. Settle yourself and then resume the exercise.

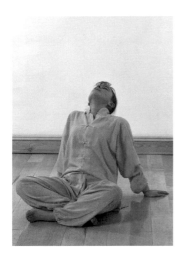

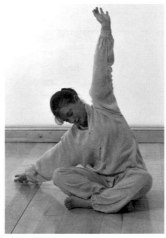

'Manifest plainness, embrace simplicity.'

TAO TEH CHING

leave you, imagine the Chi flowing freely through the joints of your upper spine, shoulders and arms. Let all the tension out of your upper body, and then from your legs, opening the joints of your lower spine, hips and knees, until you reach your feet and toes. Your whole body should now feel relaxed, but do not let your posture slump. Keep your head suspended and your back erect.

Dance Dance Dance

When your body is relaxed, return your mind to your Tan Tien. From this point on, you are free to choose your movements. You may wish to inspire yourself from the Tai Chi Form or the Chi Kung exercises, or from other forms of exercise and dance that you have taken part in; or you may want to listen to your body, and let your Chi alone guide you. This free-form meditation is particularly beneficial for those in sedentary jobs, who cannot release physical stress in their work.

209

Sitting and Standing

Still meditation is without doubt the most difficult exercise to perform. In moving meditation, your mind is centred by the gentle rhythms of your Chi, but when your body is forced to be immobile and your senses are shut off, your mind becomes bored and craves any distraction. Still meditation uses techniques to focus the mind to attain a state of inner peace. A common technique is to concentrate on your own breathing, which slows the heart and relaxes the body, while the improved flow of oxygen sharpens the mind; another is creative visualisation, in which the mind creates an imaginary place or sensation as the anchoring point of the mind.

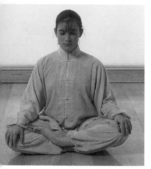

Above One of the traditional poses for yoga meditation and breathing exercises is the lotus position. In this variant, the half lotus, only one leg is held in place.

'Exhibit the unadorned and embrace the uncarved block. Have little thought of self and as few desires as possible.'

TAO TEH CHING

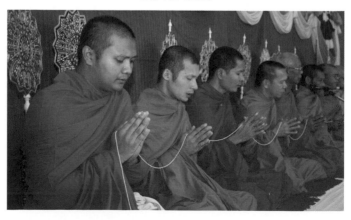

'He who conquers others has physical strength. He who conquers himself is strong.'

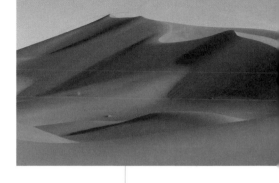

TAO TEH CHING

Sitting Meditation

If you have difficulty in sitting on the floor, you can practise meditation sitting in a chair. Do not attempt this exercise on a sofa or armchair because you will not be able to maintain the correct position of your back and head, and are more likely to fall asleep.

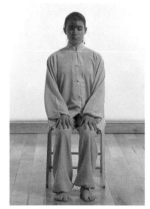

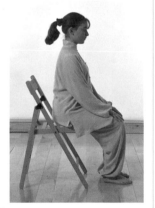

1 Sit with feet flat on the floor. Place hands on thighs and close your eyes. When you breathe in, gently contract your abdominal muscles. Hold for a count of two and breathe out.

2 Don't slump, as this will impede your breathing. Keep the mind focused on the inhalation/contraction and exhalation/relaxation. Continue for ten to twelve full breath cycles.

211

Yin and Yang Breathing

Breathing is overlooked by conventional exercise methods, which limit themselves to encouraging us to 'take a deep breath', when our lungs feel as if they're about to burst. But as the means by which our bodies obtain life-giving oxygen and expel toxins, it has long been recognised in India and China as a vital ingredient of fitness. The Indian yogic breathing techniques known as pranayama were imported to China with the Buddhist religion, and in the intervening centuries, the Chinese refined them into their own system of breathing exercises to increase health and vitality. The following two exercises will improve your breathing function and will enable you to centre your mind during meditation.

Above The Yin and Yang symbol represents the two complementary forces that make up our Universe.

1 Stand with your feet slightly apart and your arms hanging by your sides. Hold your head and upper back straight. Close your eyes if it aids your concentration. Breathe in through your nose for a count of five to eight seconds. Imagine that the air is like water being poured into a jar. Your abdomen fills first and then your chest. Hold your breath for a count of two seconds before breathing out through your mouth for a count of five to eight. Imagine that you are emptying the jar of water from the top of the chest to the bottom of your abdomen. Continue for ten to twelve full breath cycles.

2 Close your eyes and breathe out, but imagine that you are holding back half of the out-breath in your stomach. Breathe in and out again, expelling the old half of the air you held back on the previous out-breath, and taking in a new half breath of air. Continue this pattern for ten to twelve full cycles.

'The Chi
should be
excited, the
spirit should
be internally
gathered.'

Zhang Sanfeng

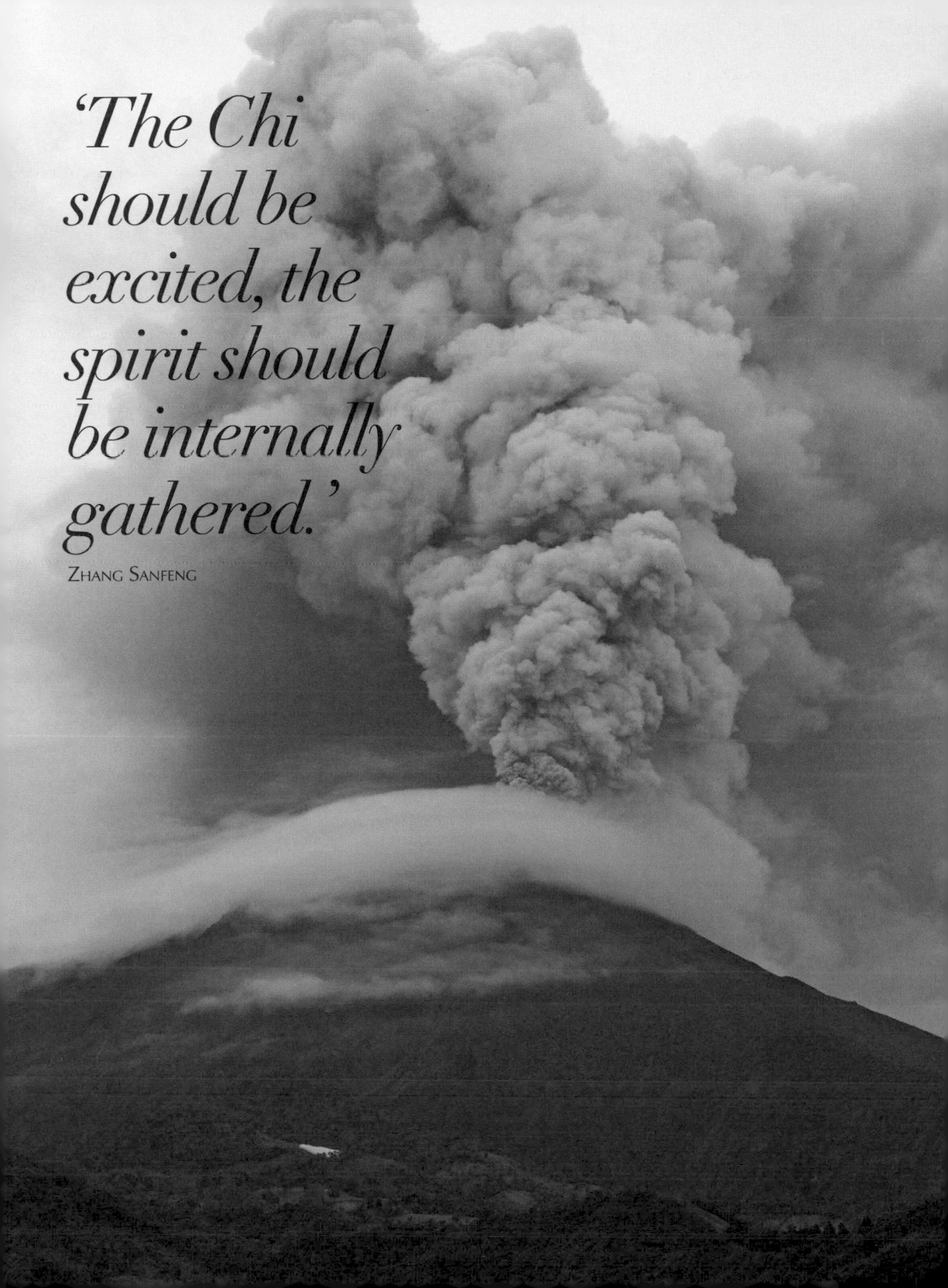

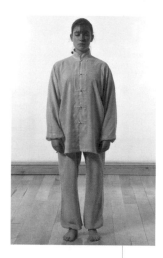

Standing – The Waterfall Method

Another technique used to centre the mind during meditation is creative visualisation. In this exercise the soothing power of water is used as the focus to aid concentration.

1 In a quiet place, stand in a relaxed stance and close your eyes. Imagine that you are standing in a shallow pool of warm water. You step under a gentle waterfall.

2 Imagine the flow of the water from your head to your shoulders, then down your chest, back and arms. Try to experience the pleasurable feeling of the water droplets on your skin, and the way they run along your limbs to your fingers and toes.

'Be as still as a mountain, move like a great river.'

WU YUXIANG

Caution

While breathing and visualisation exercises do not seem to be strenuous, they may have unexpected physical effects, such as lightheadedness and giddiness. If this happens, discontinue the exercise and sit quietly for a moment before resuming.

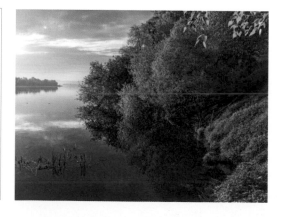

Standing Still to Keep Fit

Practice of The Form makes demands on your legs because it is performed with bent knees, which quickly tires the muscles of your hips and thighs. If the weakness of your legs is limiting the time you can spend practising, one of the easiest ways to strengthen them is by performing the standing exercises below. If you wish to practise discreetly in a queue or other public place, stand easy, hands by your side, shift your weight to one foot and bend your knees. As soon as one leg is tired, shift weight to the other foot.

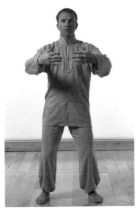
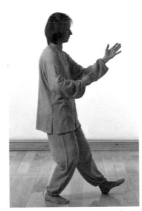
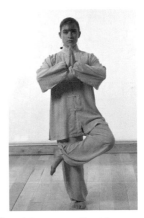

1 Stand with your feet shoulder-width apart and bend the knees. Raise both arms in front of you, keeping the elbows soft and rounded, as if you were hugging a tree. Keep your shoulders relaxed, not allowing any tension to build up in your neck and back. Feel your feet sink into the ground and become rooted, as if you were becoming part of the tree. Hold for 5 to 10 minutes.

2 Stand in the Hand Strums the Lute posture of the simplified form (see page 112). Close your eyes and hold the pose for five to ten minutes, then shake out any tension and repeat with the opposite arm and leg.

3 Helping yourself with your hands, lift your right leg and place your right foot against your left thigh. Press your palms together in front of your chest. Hold the position for five minutes and repeat with your left leg.

Conclusion

When you have reached the end of The Form, what next? Before moving to other aspects of Tai Chi, it is better to increase your skill with what you already know. Learning the sequence is relatively easy when compared to performing it correctly.

Below Practising the moves regularly is best.

The Tai Chi Master, Chen Man Ching, stated that, as he saw it, there are three important factors that one needs to become skilled in Tai Chi. These are:

(1) Practice
(2) A good teacher
(3) Natural ability

Practice is the most important of the three factors. We all have the ability to achieve good levels of success with Tai Chi, provided that we are prepared to do the practice. The only real natural ability is the ability to fit some practice into your daily routine. The majority of modern people have tight daily schedules. If you find that you are enjoying Tai Chi, and want to make some real progress, you need to learn efficient ways of practising. The first thing to do is to set reasonable goals. Take small, but manageable steps. After one practice session for your Tai Chi, your skill level will not dramatically change. It is better to practise for a short time, but often, than to have long sessions infrequently. Try to find time in your day to practise, even if it is only for a quarter of an hour. This will save you from having to repeat the same adjustments and improvements time and time again.

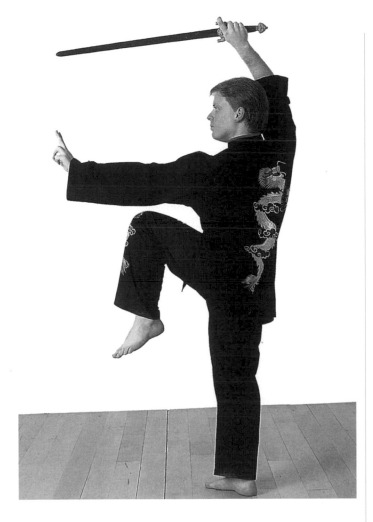

Left Weapons practice is a good next step if you wish to take your Tai Chi training further.

A successful approach is to pick out a movement and practise that particular move. You can pick any part of The Form that you like for this approach. Now practise that movement until you really know it – there are many layers of knowledge for each movement.

When you pick on a movement in this way, it will influence the whole of your Tai Chi form. You will understand the feelings behind that movement and apply them to the rest of your form without even thinking about it. This process is sometimes called

217

Right You will soon learn how effective 'softness' is against 'force'.

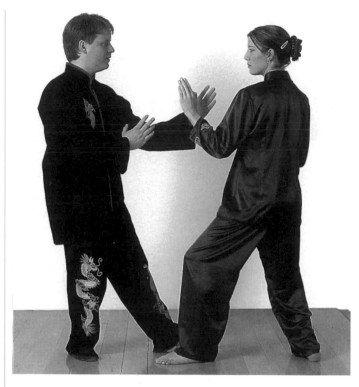

Below Learning to use a sword in Tai Chi will enhance your balance and coordination.

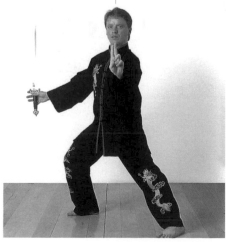

parallel learning. Working on one part in-depth will affect all of your other moves in parallel. The alternative is to work more superficially on one move after the other in a more serial approach. The serial approach is usually slower and gives less insight into the deeper aspects of Tai Chi.

Developments

You have spent some time working on the movments, so what comes next? Tai Chi encompasses many fields of knowledge. When you have a good feeling for the basics, you may wish to explore further.

A logical progression after learning the Simplified Form is to learn the traditional Yang-style form. This form contains one hundred and eight separate movements. There are, however, many repetitions of the same movements. The transitions between the moves are where work will be required. In the Simplified Form that we have learned (see pages 100–157), there are twenty-four different movements. In the traditional Yang-style Form there wil be eleven new movements to learn. Even with these new movements, the same basic energies apply. A good grounding in the Simplified Form will be priceless if you ever learn the traditional Yang form.

The lessons of Tai Chi become worthwhile when you can apply them to your daily life. The advantages of good posture are well documented and generally fairly obvious. A less obvious advantage is the idea of not using force. Aggressive situations can appear frequently, especially if you are surrounded by stress sufferers in your workplace. As a change from becoming involved with their argument cycles you may wish to use a Tai Chi approach, and let them get on with it themselves. This can save you from being drawn into their arguments, and you will be more efficient through your day and less exhausted when you get home.

Below Regular practice will deepen your understanding of Tai Chi, allowing you to 'Lift Your Spirit'.

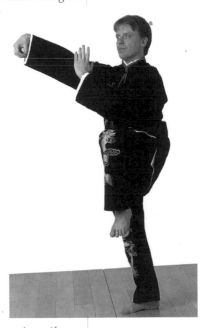

Grand Finale Finish

If Tai Chi can help you regain inner balance, it is contagious. If you have ever met a high level Tai Chi Master, you will know that they seem to exude some sort of calmness around them. If you have not met anybody like this, think about the other extreme. If you know somebody who is frequently angry, you will have seen how he or she seems to bring the anger out in other people.

So you can see that on a metaphysical level, we are affecting the Energy of the whole Universe when we practise Tai Chi. This all boils down to the most important lesson that Tai Chi or any other discipline can teach us – LIFT THE SPIRIT!

219

Resources

Finding a teacher

Now that Tai Chi is a worldwide subject, attracting more and more students looking for teachers every day, it is unfortunately necessary to start this section with a warning. Students mean money and money can mean con artists. So how do you know that a teacher is the genuine article?

After finding a teacher, try to talk to his or her pupils. What are their impressions and experiences? Is the teacher always trying to sell them books, tapes and equipment which they do not need? Is the teacher conceited and self-absorbed, always criticising other teachers? This all happens and has to be taken into account.

Of course teachers come in all psychological and physical shapes and sizes. One person may not know a great deal but may still be a good teacher. Another may know a great deal but be a poor teacher. In brief, shop around before you part with your time and money. What people learn with their first teacher tends to stick and be hard to eradicate, if it needs to be. A good rule of thumb is to find a professional Tai Chi instructor to study with. In this day and age, if a person can make a living as a Tai Chi teacher they must have a certain standard of skill and teaching ability.

Always keep your feet on the ground. Tai Chi begins and ends with the way you move and feel inside. No amount of philosophy and words can replace this. If you want to think about Tai Chi and discuss it, then you should find a Chinese philosophy seminar.

An extension of this piece of advice is that you should persevere. Learn at least one Form so you will be able to do something which has a beginning, a middle and an end. However, you may come across a teacher who emphasises correct physical movement before an entire Form is learned. This should not discourage you. It is a subject that you would have to tackle sooner or later anyway; it has just arrived sooner. If you have any doubts about your health: joints, vertebrae, heart and so forth, get a medical check-up first, or at least ask your doctor's opinion to be on the safe side. Any medical condition should be reported to your teacher before the first lesson.

More than anything, after perseverance, you will need patience and appreciation – which are closely linked. Tai Chi appreciation depends on noticing and seeing the significance of things which you might ordinarily ignore or dismiss as not worthy of attention. For example, if you occasionally notice that during your class you take a relaxed and naturally deeper breath than usual, appreciate it. It will probably be some time before your breathing deepens when doing the whole Form, but this brief experience is a taste of things to come. Then you will need patience to work and wait for it.

Facing Page and Below A teacher should find time for personal attention. A teacher should SHOW you what he wants you to do.

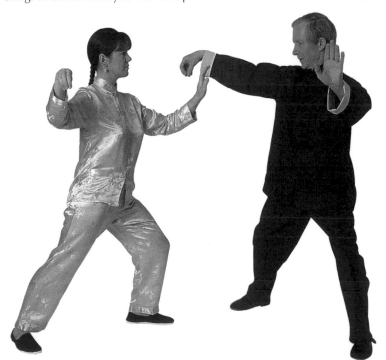

221

Index

Page numbers in **bold** refer to illustrations

Index